How to Beat Chronic Fatigue Syndrome... and Get Your Life Back!

Warren Tattersall & Helene Malmsio

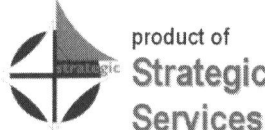

product of
Strategic Services

How to Beat Chronic Fatigue Syndrome… and Get Your Life Back!

Copyright © 2012 by Warren Tattersall & Helene Malmsio. All rights reserved worldwide.

No part of this book may be reproduced by any photographic, xerographic, digital or electronic means except for purposes of review without the prior written permission of the copyright holder.

Publisher: Helene Malmsio & Strategic Services
PO Box 412, Maryborough, Victoria, Australia 3465

http://www.learn-how-to-do-it.com and
http://www.thehealthsuccesssite.com

This publication is designed to provide accurate and authoritative information in regard to the subject matter covered. It is sold the understanding that the publisher is not engaged in rendering legal, accounting, or other professional services. If legal advice or other expert assistance is required, the services of a competent professional person should be sought.

First Printing, 2012, 2nd Edition 2014

Revised 2014

ISBN-13: 978-1503315808
ISBN-10: 1503315800

Printed in the United States of America

No Liability

The information and resources in this book are not intended to be a substitute for professional advice. While all attempts have been made to verify the information provided in this publication, neither the author nor the publisher assumes any responsibility for errors, omissions or contrary interpretation of the subject matter herein.

There is no guarantee of validity of accuracy of any content. Any perceived slight of specific people or organizations is unintentional. This book and its creators are not responsible for the content of any sites linked to from it.

Under no circumstances will the product creator or any of the distributors of this product, be liable to any party for any direct, indirect, punitive, special, incidental, or other consequential damages arising directly or indirectly from the use of this product. This product is provided "as is" and without warranties.

Use of this product indicates your acceptance of the "No Liability" policy. If you do not agree with our "No Liability" policy, then you are not permitted to use or distribute this product (if applicable.)

Failure to read this notice in its entirety does not void your agreement to this policy should you decide to use this product. Applicable law may not allow the limitation or exclusion of liability or incidental or consequential damages, so the above limitation or exclusion may not apply to you.

The liability for damages, regardless of the form of the action, shall not exceed the actual fee paid for the product.

Table of Contents

What is Chronic Fatigue Syndrome? 1

    Symptoms of Chronic Fatigue Syndrome 4

    Impact on Your Life 7

    Outlook for Chronic Fatigue Syndrome 9

    Becoming Your Own Advocate 10

Chronic Fatigue Syndrome through the Years 13

    A Changing Diagnosis 13

    Lake Tahoe Cluster 14

    The Yuppie Flu 14

    What's in a Name? 15

    Looking for Cause 15

    Can I Beat a Disease that Has No Cure? 17

What Causes CFS? 21

    A Healthy Defense 21

    The Immune System Players 21

    The important cells of the immune system include: 22

    Removing Toxins 23

    Why Do We Seem to Be Inundated with Health Problems? 24

    The Body Breakdown and Chronic Fatigue Syndrome 29

    Don't Dwell on Past Mistakes 30

Do I Have Chronic Fatigue Syndrome? 33
What Could Be Wrong? 33
More than One Problem at a Time 35
Do You Have Risk Factors? 35
Fear is the Enemy 36
Preparing for Your Visit to the Doctor 37
At Your Appointment 38
Does Your Doctor Understand and Treat Chronic Fatigue Syndrome? 40

Lifestyle Changes that Can Improve CFS 43
Pacing Therapy 44
Diet & Nutrition for Beating CFS 55
Nutritional Supplementation 59
Exercise 66
Detoxification 68
Probiotics 72
Keep Candida in Check 72
The Restorative Power of Sleep 73
Guard Your Energy Reserves 74
Avoid Addictive Habits 76

Medical Treatment for Chronic Fatigue Syndrome 79
Antidepressants 79
Anti-Inflammatories 80

    Sleeping Medication 80

    CBT - Cognitive Behavioral Therapy 81

    Why Does This Cognitive Behavioral Therapy Work? 87

    Remember that CFS Is Not Like Other Health Conditions 88

    Seek Support When Trying Out Cognitive Behavioral Therapy 88

Complementary Therapies to Manage CFS 91

    Chinese Medicine 91

    Massage Therapy 92

    Physical Therapy 93

    Energy Medicine 93

    Chiropractic Care 94

    Homeopathy 95

    Aromatherapy 95

    Dietitian 96

Rebounding from Relapses 97

    Be Aware of Your Cycles 97

    Two Steps Forward, One Step Back 98

    Triggers for Relapse 98

    An Opportunity to Grow 99

    Be Your Own Champion 100

Supporting Someone with CFS 101

    What You Need to Know 101

How CFS Can Affect a Caregiver 103

Tips for Caregivers 104

Be Kind and Forgiving of Yourself and Others 108

Putting It All Together 109

Be Willing to Try New Things 109

Don't Put Pressure On Yourself 109

Don't Delay 110

Remember That Things Will Get Better 110

What is Chronic Fatigue Syndrome?

Chronic Fatigue Syndrome (CFS) was once not very well known, though many people probably suffered from it there was no medical explanation for it and many sufferers were considered to be 'slackers', hypochondriacs and malingerers. In modern times we have a better understanding of this difficult health problem.

Although the actual causes for chronic fatigue syndrome are not currently known, scientists, doctors and researchers around the world believe that this condition can be related to high levels of stress and lifestyle factors caused by viral infection, a malfunction of the immune system, and that it can have a genetic component as well.

We would go further than that and put into this discussion that modern living and the pressures we put ourselves under can damage our body's ability to ingest nutrition so that we do not absorb much of the nutrition from what we eat and on a cellular level are literally starving to death in the midst of plenty.

But no matter the cause, this can be a debilitating illness that isn't always understood well by those who have it and often understood even less by the people who love and care for them. If you have CFS, or you think you have it, it's important to understand some basic information about it.

It's also important to know modern medicine and healthcare and even alternate health practitioners treat CFS as a disease and that there are many ways CFS can be treated, though there is currently no standard or single specific 'cure' as such. Knowledge is power, and the more you know the better you'll be able to manage your health.

When you're feeling exhausted all the time and have some of the symptoms listed in this chapter, you may think that you have a passing illness. In fact, you could be right about that. As the symptoms begin to intrude more and more upon your life there comes a point where you feel that something has to be wrong but you may still be hesitant to talk to your doctor about it. You may fear you have a serious health condition or if your symptoms are still somewhat under control you may fear your doctor will think it's all in your head.

But it's important not to neglect your health and not to let your symptoms be swept under the rug. It's always best to confront the health problems sooner rather than later and determine a course of treatment or management.

In this book you'll learn about the basics of chronic fatigue syndrome, how it's diagnosed, and how it's treated. You'll also learn how to manage your life so that you can continue to do the things you enjoy.

We have each experienced more than 30 years of CFS and have tried and tested many recommended therapies and remedies over those years. Some did not work, but some did.

Perplexingly, we have come across many people with CFS who found that something worked very well for them but that very same approach would have little or no benefit for others.

There is such a variation of severity in the way different people experience CFS and in the treatments that different people find effective in dealing with it that we have written this comprehensive book as the first step in helping others to learn from our trials of popular therapies.

This is not a clinical document or a medical paper. We will not be delivering hundreds of pages of research results from Clinics or Universities. There are already so many sources online where you can read the latest studies on this subject, along with all the forums established to discuss and review the newest fashionable 'treatments' and fads being talked about.

What we have done in this book is not to talk about dry facts and statistics, or theorizing the pros and cons of untried and unproven 'cures'. Instead we present the strategies and therapies for CFS that we have been using and sharing for 20 years, to show you how to start taking control of your condition right now and reclaim your life again.

If you are already exhausted, depressed, confused and totally overwhelmed by the frustrating amount of information out there about CFS and ME and Fibromyalgia and related illnesses, you are not likely to want to have to plow through even more facts and statistics in this book that can't show you how to start improving your health today anyway.

We are giving you tools to be able to confirm if your symptoms match the common CFS indicators so, if they do, you can get on with the job of beating your chronic fatigue!

This book is written to help you review the therapies that have already worked for others, make your selection of what resonates with your condition and lifestyle, and translate those strategies into your own individual therapy plan.

Although we are not medical practitioners, we have had decades of experience in sharing our personal experiences toward helping other people to deal with their CFS symptoms as well.

In summary, our focus it to give you strategies in this book that will allow you to explain what it is that you are dealing with to the friends and family who surround you, give you tools to help deal with your condition, empower you to know how to reach out for professional guidance and support and, ultimately, you will be able to get a lot of relief from your condition.

Symptoms of Chronic Fatigue Syndrome

Before we talk about how we can overcome chronic fatigue syndrome, we need to talk about what it is specifically and how we can recognize it in ourselves and others.

It is true that everyone gets tired sometimes. We perform physical and mental activity that causes us to be exhausted and even unable to function in some cases.

But if you suffer from chronic fatigue syndrome, you feel like that all the time, even if you haven't necessarily done any unusual activities that might have caused you to get really tired in the first place. Simply speaking, with this disorder, you get tired for almost no reason, and you stay tired.

People that have CFS report of not being able to function normally, as well as feeling pain, experiencing loss of memory, being unable to concentrate, of not being able to sleep and of not being refreshed even when they do get some sleep.

A typical scenario is a lady with mild CFS who said that she used to go shopping and come home and put the shopping away and then sit down and have a cup of tea.

As her condition worsened she found that she would do her shopping and then immediately have to sit and have a cup of tea, and rest for quite a while, before she had the energy to even begin putting away the shopping.

She knew something was wrong but did not know what it was, and was looking for answers to her unexplained increase in daily tiredness. The hardest thing for her was that she could not find anyone who understood what she was dealing with. If you have some issues and are not sure how to begin to deal then then hopefully we can help you.

Unfortunately, it is not currently possible to medically determine any one factor that can be identified as causing CFS. There appears to be a wide range of triggers that can be responsible. What is more, it is difficult to diagnose it, because many of the other diseases people suffer from can also cause tiredness and fatigue as one of their symptoms.

In order to help people identify CFS, experts in that field have gathered and indicated a few symptoms that an individual has to suffer from if they are to be diagnosed as having CFS.

Most of those symptoms are common for other diseases as well, but if you have four or more of them all at once, and have had them consistently for a considerable amount of time, and also suffer from chronic fatigue at the same time, then chances are you have the syndrome.

The range of common symptoms includes:

1. **Tiredness.** As we mentioned before, everyone gets tired, but what we mean here is being very tired for more than 24 hours after performing physical activities.

    If you are tired when you wake up and even a long sleep does not seem to refresh you, if you regularly find that you lose concentration, like if in the middle of the afternoon you try to read something and then read it again, but it just does not sink in to your brain.

This is also often described by sufferers as a feeling of "brain fog" where you are so exhausted that you just cannot concentrate or stay focused, and develop a poor memory.

Tiredness like this that stays with you weeks or months at a time is the sort of tiredness associated with CFS.

2. **Headaches.** This relates mostly to headaches that you haven't had before or different types of headaches from what you would normally experience.

For instance if your headache is very strong or it occurs much more frequently than usual, it is possible that you are suffering from the syndrome.

3. **Lack of sleep.** If you have trouble sleeping at night and when you do sleep it is not refreshing so you wake feeling tired before you even begin your day, then that is an indicator many people with CFS suffer from.

Especially if you are exhausted when you go to bed, but despite this you experience insomnia and still can't get to sleep.

4. **Pain in your muscles.** If you have pain in your muscles that you have not experienced before, and it does not go away after you rest, that is a warning sign.

5. **Chronic sore throat.** Another symptom of CFS is a constantly sore throat. Now, obviously we don't mean your throat just hurting a little bit. Rather, this is an unusual pain in your throat that lasts for days, weeks or even months.

Of course, all of the above symptoms may also happen if you suffer from a different disease. That is why you need to have at least four of those to be diagnosed with CFS. And other conditions must be ruled out by your medical doctor.

There are also other symptoms that CFS patients have reported suffering from. They are less frequent than the ones mentioned above; nevertheless it is important for you to learn what they are and consider if they have been or are affecting you now:

- Intolerance for alcohol.
- Dryness of mouth and eyes.
- Chronic diarrhea.
- Chronic cough.
- Irregular heartbeat.
- Sweating at night.
- Pain in your jaw.
- Abnormal weight loss.
- Constantly feeling nauseous.
- Being dizzy all the time.
- Experiencing shortness of breath.

In addition, there may be other symptoms that are individual to you. In this book we will talk about natural methods of getting your life back as well as some supplements and medications you can use in your therapy.

Impact on Your Life

When it comes to having CFS, there's a wide range of experiences. If your symptoms are in the milder range you may be able to continue with many of your normal activities even though you might find it difficult just living your life day by day. However, in severe cases that isn't so as life can totally fall apart around you.

Many people who have severe chronic fatigue syndrome symptoms are unable to any longer handle their daily responsibilities at work or at home, or both. In fact, some people experience such problems that they remain bedridden for most of the time and can't do much of anything for many months or even years.

As you can imagine, this impacts not only you but your family and friends. You may suffer from memory and attention deficit problems as well as a growing depression as your condition lingers on. The activities and chores that you can no longer do yourself are often transferred to other family members.

Very often the condition also leads to food intolerance and food allergies. Celiac disease for example is quite common with people who have a more severe CFS.

Some people become sensitive to chemicals in the environment and react badly to aerosol sprays, to perfumes, even to cleaning products and other environment chemicals that most people just do not notice.

Fortunately, there's much you can do to promote wellness and to get back to many of your daily activities.

You must learn the fundamentals of your own best self care and start to be kind to yourself to support your body's healing and wellness journey.

It's also important for your caregivers, friends, and family members to become educated about CFS as it will also impact their lives. It's important for them to understand that you have a real health problem and learn how to support you in your recovery process.

Caregivers must also learn to support their own wellness and not become drained by new responsibilities. That can be difficult to do, but through education and support caregivers can get relief from the burden they carry themselves in supporting someone who has CFS. We will discuss these strategies as well further along in here.

Chronic fatigue syndrome isn't an imaginary illness. Many people describe the symptoms as similar to the flu. If you've ever had the flu you know that it feels so wretched you almost wish for someone to put you out of your misery.

But with CFS you feel like you have the flu all the time. And instead of being able to call in sick to work you most likely have to find a way to just keep going. People look at you and think you look well enough, so you must be okay.

When you feel so badly and no one understands it, you can feel even worse about the situation. Many people end up losing their jobs, friends, sometimes their spouses, and even relationships with close family members because of this illness.

CFS is unlike the flu though, in that it is not contagious. It is your problem and you have to live with it but at least there is not a concern about other people catching it from you.

And while it was once very poorly understood, the medical community is finally acknowledging this syndrome exists and more research is being conducted to look for a cause and cure.

Outlook for Chronic Fatigue Syndrome

Some people with chronic fatigue syndrome have the symptoms for six months to a year and then return to their normal energy levels. However, more than half of the people who have been diagnosed with it still feel symptoms many years later.

And you may have symptoms for a block of time followed by relief only to experience a relapse of the condition down the road. Because chronic fatigue syndrome is an individual experience, it's impossible to say what your particular outlook will be.

However, we do know that people who have a good management plan and stick to it have better quality of life and can actually return to many of their normal activities. That's good news for you!

Becoming Your Own Advocate

When it comes to your health, the more you know the better you can make good health decisions. Doctors are notoriously busy people who sometimes make assumptions about what you know or don't know.

It's important for you to take charge of your own health. If you have a good doctor who is genuinely interested in your health and your condition then you can work in partnership with them and other health professionals and truly advocate for what's best for your own body and life.

People who are intimidated by 'authority figures' like doctors, or don't feel confident enough to speak up and ask questions for clarification from specialists should ask a friend or family member to attend appointments with them as their Advocate and speak on their behalf and take notes for them, if necessary.

It is important that you get into the driver's seat and control your own recovery process. Do not let yourself be pushed into taking prescription medication or testing remedies that you are not absolutely certain are suitable for you.

With this book, you'll get information that can help you to feel confident about asking questions and truly participating in your own treatment and management of chronic fatigue syndrome.

Having a solid foundation on which to build your understanding of CFS is critical to beating this health condition and feeling your best.

Obviously, we want you to understand that you can always contact us if you have any questions. We will be more than happy to help you with anything you need.

Chronic Fatigue Syndrome through the Years

Chronic fatigue syndrome seems like a relatively new condition. But even though it hasn't had its name for very long, CFS has probably been around for hundreds of years. In early medicine it was thought to be a psychiatric disorder.

A Changing Diagnosis

George Miller Beard, a notable neurologist in the 1800s was known for his discovery and treatment of a disorder called neurasthenia, which was characterized by fatigue, headaches, anxiety, and depression.

This diagnosis was very popular for a time. It was seen as a problem with behavior and psychology rather than having any sort of physical cause. This was the diagnosis given to those who experienced these symptoms but didn't have any sort of infection.

However, as medicine became more advanced this particular diagnosis fell out of favor and is no longer used. In the mid-1900s, some other conditions were suspected to be related to these symptoms.

In 1938 one doctor, Alexander Gillia, believed the symptoms to be related to polio and called the syndrome atypical poliomyelitis when he worked with patients in Los Angeles. Over the next 20 years similar diagnoses were made all over the world.

This group of symptoms was thought to mimic polio, though it wasn't truly polio. This mysterious illness plagued people in Switzerland, Australia, South Africa, the United States, as well as many others.

Throughout the 20th century various doctors tried to attribute causes and develop diagnoses for this group of symptoms. But it wasn't until the 1980s that chronic fatigue syndrome was attributed to these patterns.

Lake Tahoe Cluster

In the 1980s a cluster of people reported symptoms that we now attribute to CFS. At that time it was believed that they had been exposed to the Epstein-Barr virus and that they were suffering from long-term effects of infection.

This syndrome was called Chronic Epstein-Barr Virus, but was also known as "Raggedy Ann Syndrome" because if the fatigue that was the hallmark of the illness.

While this was believed to be the cause, a group of researchers later found it not to be the cause.

Those in the cluster were tested and found not to have been exposed to Epstein-Barr. At this time, in 1988, the term "chronic fatigue syndrome" was coined to describe the condition and that term is still in use today.

The Yuppie Flu

It's been a difficult struggle for people with CFS to be seen as people with legitimate health problems. In the 80s, chronic fatigue syndrome was also called the "yuppie flu" or the "shirker's disease".

People who had the symptoms of fatigue, headaches, muscle pain, and sore throat were thought to be trying to get out of actually working. Since there was no medical sounding diagnosis, the condition must have been all in their heads.

It took until 1999 for the United States Centers for Disease Control to acknowledge that this is a real medical condition and allocate money for research and awareness. This has helped to legitimize chronic fatigue syndrome.

What's in a Name?

Perhaps one of the most frustrating problems with CFS is its given name. Because it sounds like a layperson description many people don't take it seriously. There have been many people who have suggested that the name ought to be changed to give medical legitimacy.

For example, some people would prefer to use the name similar to what was used in Britain to describe the disease: myalgic encephalopathy. This is a general term for muscle pain and inflammation of the nervous system.

The idea is that a more medical sounding name will naturally allow people to take the illness more seriously. In the future, it would not be surprising if the name were to become more scientific sounding.

Looking for Cause

In the years since this illness was termed 'Chronic Fatigue Syndrome', researchers have stopped looking at psychological problems and depression as the cause. It's generally believed that this is a true physiological condition.

However, no one is really sure of the cause. Many researchers have looked for a common viral cause, but no study has been successful at delivering results that could be repeated.

In the authors opinions there are a range of causes that can be the main contributing factor in difference cases. That opinion has its foundation in personal experience in working with the condition, and from working with people who have the condition, and it is not scientifically based.

We will discuss these views with you through this book as among the many ways of understanding the condition and include our own experience of ways to approach dealing with the condition.

The good news is that there are millions of dollars allocated for research for this illness and new developments are possible. Scientists are hard at work looking for any type of cause they can find.

Research is still being conducted to look for one single cause, but until such research proves to be successful the current medical community focuses on managing the symptoms rather than curing them.

In our own experience we believe that there are a range of conditions that precede the onset of CFS.

There is a group of people who have had issues with low energy, lack of stamina, allergies, and immune system problems for a long time. In some cases this has been that way for as long as they can remember. When the condition turns around, like it did for Warren (co-author of this book) it is like a complete change of life.

Many people who suffer from CFS have indeed had a viral condition previously. Normally that turns out to have been 6 to 12 months or so prior to the first real symptoms of CFS appearing.

Others can point to a time of high stress and pressure in their lives: sometimes work related, maybe they have been working as a

Career for someone who has been ill for some time, or a relationship breakup, or as a result of conditions in their life that have been stressful and has left them tired and run down.

Then there is normally a trigger event, normally one that involves the use of antibiotics, and they begin down the path towards CFS.

Finally we come across the people who have been exposed to chemicals or have had long term substance abuse. This is a group that has a much harder time recovering from CFS but they also, in time, can overcome their problems.

Can I Beat a Disease that Has No Cure?

At this point you may be wondering if it's possible to beat chronic fatigue syndrome. After all, this is an illness that doesn't have a known cause or cure in the medical community.

While that may seem discouraging, it's important to take heart. There really is good news when it comes to chronic fatigue syndrome.

The authors have worked with dozens and dozens of people who have had CFS and who are now back to normal and productive lives. The issue with CFS is that there are no tests to specifically show that you have CFS and so by definition there is no test to show you are cured.

When you find the method that works for you then you will need to monitor your own health and keep focused on the time when you can live a normal life again.

In the last few decades there has been much improvement in what we do understand about CFS.

We now know:

- More about how the immune system works and how to protect the body from harm
- How malabsorption of nutrients and lack of correct nutrition in your diet can have a direct impact on long term health
- How changes in our environment and society can contribute to the greater number of health problems, specifically chronic diseases, that we experience
- Medications that can help to relieve symptoms and improve quality of life
- How nutrition can have a direct impact on turning around CFS
- Lifestyle changes that can relieve symptoms and help you to cope with energy ebbs and flows
- Practices in complementary medicine that can relieve inflammation and restore good health
- How to talk to people about this illness so they can understand it as a "real" medical problem
- How to find others with CFS and seek support

Don't let the fact that Western medicine hasn't offered a cure for CFS make you feel there is no hope for a joyful and active life again.

There's much you can do in partnership with a physician or complementary medical provider to improve your condition. You can also take many steps in your own lifestyle that will help you to have relief from your CFS symptoms and improve your life.

It's important not to be discouraged or to give up – you have more power than you know to keep chronic fatigue syndrome from defining who you are.

What Causes CFS?

While there's no one specific cause that's been isolated for chronic fatigue syndrome, there are many suspects. It's important for you to understand what may be contributing to your condition in order to have the wellness you desire.

But before we look at what be causing the malfunction in your body, let's look at how your body fights disease in general. This can give you insight into some of the symptoms you're experiencing.

A Healthy Defense

Your body has a range of natural mechanisms in place to keep you healthy. The immune system is possibly the most highly sophisticated tool you have to stay healthy. It's also extremely complicated.

There's no need to get too technical here, but it will help you to have a basic understanding of how your body keeps you from getting sick when things are working the way they should.

The Immune System Players

Your body's immune system is made up of organs and cells that do the job of keeping out foreign invaders and destroying the ones that make it into the body. The first line of defense for the body is your skin.

Your skin is a protective covering that makes it difficult for pathogens to get into the body. However, you have thinner tissue that is vulnerable in the eyes, mouth, nose, anus, and genital areas. These are the most likely places of disease to enter the body.

You also have a breach of security in the skin when you have a wound, cut, or burn that allows bacteria, viruses, and fungi to enter in. Keeping skin healthy through good hygiene and good nutrition can help you stay well.

Your bones are also an essential component of the immune system. Inside the bones is softer tissue called bone marrow. This is where most of your blood cells are produced, including many of the white blood cells that make up your immune system.

The thymus is a gland in the body that works to mature white cells produced in the bone marrow. It's responsible for producing T cells, cells that help to coordinate immune response and actually kill some pathogens.

The spleen is another important organ of the immune system. This is a place where the immune cells are filtered. Old cells are destroyed and new cells become activated in this organ.

The lymph nodes are also important players in the immune system. These glands are responsible for filtering immune cells and pathogens from the fluid in the body called lymph. Then the filtered fluid is returned to circulate throughout the body.

The important cells of the immune system include:

- Helper T-Cells – their primary job is to alert the immune system that there's a foreign invader after getting information from other cells

- Killer T-Cells – these cells kill cells in the body that have been infected with a pathogen

- B Cells – produce antibodies for the specific foreign invader that is attacking

- Phagocytes – these are cells that eat foreign invaders or injured cells

Basically, when a foreign invader is noticed by the body, the cells of the immune system kick into high gear producing antibodies and destroying the pathogens and cells infected by them.

It can also remember enemies from the past so that if they return, the immune response can be much faster the second time. That's why many illnesses only have to be experienced once before you become immune. The next time your body can wipe out the invader quickly and easily.

Removing Toxins

In addition to fighting bacteria, viruses, and fungi your body also gets invaded by toxins. But it has mechanisms for removing those toxins from the body. The main job of this goes to the liver.

The liver actually filters out toxins from alcohol, medications, and other substances that make their way into your body. It also helps to get rid of the waste that your body makes as a natural process.

Some waste gets transferred to the fluid made by the liver called bile. That bile then goes to the digestive system and leaves the body as solid waste. Excess bile that's produced is stored in the gall bladder to be used later.

Other wastes travel through the blood to the kidneys where they are removed in the urine. The adrenal glands located at the top of the kidneys are responsible for producing hormones to regulate the body.

There seems to be a group of CFS sufferers who can trace their condition back to chemical contamination. This is something that can be addressed by dietary and nutritional processes and so can be cleared up.

If this is your situation then you will have to get the toxins out of your body and, in the process, you are going to again suffer the effects of having these chemicals loose in your system. It is a challenging thing to do and you can expect the spend 90 days dealing with these effects as you detoxify the initial flush of chemicals from your body,

Why Do We Seem to Be Inundated with Health Problems?

One would think that with advances in medical technology, we would be healthier than ever. And while some diseases have been completely eradicated or have at least been treated in ways they can be cured, we have more chronic disease than ever before.

The diseases such as smallpox, polio, and scarlet fever that were once the culprits of high mortality rates in populations have been eliminated or cured. Now the big killers are heart disease and diabetes.

While medical advances and public health measures have given us the capability of being healthier than ever, we find that our environment and lifestyle are contributing to many of the health problems we face today.

Talking with a specialist doctor recently he said that there are people he sees who have very rare diseases that few people in the medical profession have seen in their local areas.

He then said that people having rare diseases are becoming very common. What he was saying is that medical science has become very good at identifying what is wrong with people but that our whole society is producing more and more people who are unwell with rare diseases.

We are suffering rare health problems and the instance of individuals having such conditions seems to increase in direct relationship to the wealth that we create and the lifestyle choices that come into our lives.

Many believe that the further our society moves from 'natural' foods and balanced, low stress, lifestyles the more common will be people with general health problems and with problems that are unusual and difficult to identify.

In addition to these rare health conditions there are other conditions that are also very serious but which are clearly lifestyle based and that are becoming so common that society is starting to accept as being somewhat normal.

This is often related to poor dietary choices. With over 50% of adults in many western countries now being overweight the flow on effect is that lifestyle diseases like diabetes are now at epidemic proportions in first and second world countries.

In 1984, the U.S. Department of Health and Human Services said that if Americans ate less fat and more fiber, cases of colon cancer in the United States could fall by 30 percent. Nowadays many medical authorities estimate that a much higher percentage of bowel cancer could be avoided by having regular exercise and more fiber in your diet. The point here is that lifestyle and diet have a direct impact upon our health.

These factors may also be directly related to the problem of CFS.

Let's take a look at some of the common contributors to our poor state of health that can lead to problems such as chronic fatigue syndrome.

Stress

Stress is a huge factor in the breakdown of our bodies. We are moving at a faster pace than ever before and the pressures of finances, appointments, and other worries can leave us feeling broken down.

Stress also contributes to other unhealthy lifestyle behaviors such as lack of sleep, substance abuse, and poor diet.

Diet

The modern diet has become full of processed foods with lots of sugar, saturated fats, and artificial ingredients.

In addition, many people don't get enough of the good stuff such as fruits, vegetables, protein, and whole grains that keep the body fed good nutrients.

Most modern western diets have lower levels of protein than is recommended to maintain a healthy weight.

Medical advice across the board says that we should be eating at least 5 portions of fruit and vegetables a day and yet studies constantly show that actual consumption is generally well below the recommended level.

People also eat larger portion sizes than they did even two or three decades ago which further contributes to problems such as obesity and diabetes.

In other words, we're getting too much of the bad stuff and not enough of the good stuff in our diets.

Sedentary Lifestyle

We have many modern conveniences that make work easier for us. But they also contribute to the sedentary lifestyle many of us live.

Instead of spending our time plowing the fields or making everything from scratch, we spend our days at desks typing on computers.

Many researchers argue that the lack of physical activity in developed nations contributes more to the obesity problem than the poor diet we eat.

Our bodies were made to move and when we deprive them of that opportunity, the systems break down.

Environmental Toxins

In an industrialized society, one of the least desirable outcomes is that we have more waste and toxicity in the environment. This could be pollution of the air, the soil, or the water.

The toxins that make their way into our environment also make their way into our food supply and air supply. We come in contact with many chemicals that aren't good for the body on a daily basis.

Lack of Sleep

Sleep is an essential healing mechanism built into the body. But you probably wouldn't be too surprised to hear that most people don't get enough of it. We need about 10 hours of uninterrupted sleep each day.

But because of all the technology we have that allows us to stay up late working on computers, watching television, and even just reading by lamplight we often get far fewer than 10 hours, often surviving on 6 hours or less sleep most work days.

Too Little Water

Most people drink too little water.

Hydration levels in women should be 45 to 60% and men 50 to 65%. A very large portion of people have hydration levels lower than this and are dehydrated.

This makes it a lot harder for your body to work efficiently and to flush out environmental toxins and poisons.

Over Medication

Another problem we have in our culture is that we tend to be overmedicated for illness. Infections that could probably run their course naturally are often treated with antibiotics.

And improper adherence to the prescription instructions often causes problems.

For example, many people stop taking their antibiotics when their symptoms improve rather than finishing the course. This leads to the development of drug resistant pathogens that are difficult to treat.

Mobile Society

With the convenience of worldwide air travel, people are constantly moving all over the globe. Bacteria, viruses, and other pathogens can take a free trip to anywhere in the world in just a matter of days.

That makes it more likely to be exposed to diseases that were once found in global pockets.

An example of this is how we now face risk of deadly influenza strains from overseas that years ago would not have reached our borders.

Substance Use/Abuse

You also need to factor in lifestyle choices such as drinking alcohol, taking illicit medications, and using tobacco products in the decline of our general health.

These substances are often taken to alleviate stress or emotional and physical pain, only to leave the user feeling worse than he did before he started.

And these behaviors are putting toxins directly into your body that can lead to illness.

The Body Breakdown and Chronic Fatigue Syndrome

It's important to recognize that your lifestyle factors as well as those in the world at large could contribute to the problems leading to chronic fatigue syndrome.

That said, it's not helpful or healthy to dwell on blaming yourself for the illness you now face.

Many scientists believe that there is a specific virus that could be the cause of the symptoms experienced with CFS. Perhaps you've encountered a virus that has lingering effects.

But even if one specific virus is identified, it's unlikely that the discovery will provide a cure for chronic fatigue.

Instead, for now, it's important to realize that you need to do the very best you can to support your body in developing a healthy immune system and do everything you possibly can to avoid taxing it with too many toxins.

And, if you're reading this because you're interested in preventing chronic fatigue syndrome, the best thing you can do is make choices that will keep your immune system as strong as possible and avoid substances that can cause your body to have to go into overdrive with toxin filtering.

Even a healthy person who's deprived of sleep, fed a junk diet, inundated with stress and toxins, and exposed to resilient viruses will become unhealthy very fast. It's important to see how lifestyle and wellness are connected.

We will discuss lifestyle in greater detail in chapter 5. At this point it's important for you to understand that there may be parts of your lifestyle that have opened you up to this illness.

Don't Dwell on Past Mistakes

But don't beat yourself up! Many people feel like they must have done something to deserve feeling so badly and that simply isn't true. Instead of focusing on all that you've done incorrectly, focus on what you will do from now on.

And remember that coming in contact with viruses and environmental toxins has very little to do with conscious choices on your part. The problems with diet and exercise are personal choices, but they're heavily influenced by the norms of our society.

In order to beat chronic fatigue syndrome you'll need to change your perspective about the way you handle health problems. Often we go to the doctor expecting to come out with a cure.

Unfortunately with chronic fatigue syndrome that just isn't an option. There's definitely medical help available, but much of what needs to be done is really about changing your lifestyle (as is the case with many health conditions).

In this book you'll get many tools that can help you to feel better and experience wellness. As you read, think about how you'll implement these tools.

Otherwise they'll just sit in the toolbox gathering dust instead of working hard for you to heal.

Do I Have Chronic Fatigue Syndrome?

When you're not feeling well, an appointment with the doctor can make a bad situation even more stressful. But you don't have to feel intimidated or worried when you go to the doctor with the proper preparation.

In this chapter you'll learn how to document your symptoms and which questions you need to ask at your appointment. You'll also learn how you can find a doctor who knows how to work with someone who has chronic fatigue syndrome.

What Could Be Wrong?

As was mentioned earlier, the symptoms of CFS are also shared by many other illnesses. So while you might think you have chronic fatigue syndrome, it may actually be something else lurking in your system.

It's important to have a thorough examination to rule out other possibilities and to be very clear about the symptoms you're experiencing. The more detail you can give your doctor, the better.

Some possible causes of your symptoms could include:

- Fibromyalgia
- Depression
- Viral, bacterial, or fungal infection
- Environmental toxin exposure
- Obesity
- Sleep disorders
- Iron deficiency anemia

- Hypothyroidism
- Hormonal imbalances
- Side effects from medications
- Heart defect or disease
- Irritable bowel syndrome
- Overgrowth of systemic yeast
- Excess caffeine use
- Substance abuse
- Some cancers

This list is by no means exhaustive. But when all of these are ruled out by medical testing and careful attention to your symptoms, you're left with the possibility of chronic fatigue syndrome.

As you go through this list do not get the impression that all of these things are separate. If you have CFS then you can expect that you will have Iron deficiency anemia or some other food allergies.

If you have CSF then you can expect your immune system to be low so viral, bacterial, or fungal infection may be attacking you regularly. You may have Irritable bowel syndrome or overgrowth of systemic yeast.

What we were saying is that if the doctor identifies any of these problems in your health test then think about how they relate to the symptoms of CFS.

This is the sort of thing that makes it so difficult to identify CFS and for medical professionals to be able to prescribe something to deal with the problem.

More than One Problem at a Time

It's also possible that you have chronic fatigue syndrome along with an overlapping condition. It's not uncommon for people to have more than one culprit contributing to their symptoms.

For example, fibromyalgia and CFS often go hand in hand. There's also a condition called multiple chemical sensitivity (MCS) that is frequently found together with CFS. This is a condition where exposure to a specific chemical causes symptoms to be exacerbated.

It's also common for mental health problems to go hand in hand with CFS. For example, there's a higher rate of depression and eating disorders in people who have chronic fatigue syndrome. However, it's not clear if this is caused by CFS or not.

Irritable bowel syndrome, chronic problems with headache and ADHD are also found in higher numbers in the population of people with chronic fatigue syndrome. It's just important to be aware that your CFS may not be the only problem and you may have to deal with and treat a number of different health conditions.

Do You Have Risk Factors?

Because there is no one single known cause of chronic fatigue, only study of the populations of people with CFS can give us some idea of the most common risk factors. Some people do seem to be more likely to develop the syndrome than others.

Women seem to be more at risk for CFS as four out of five cases occur in women. However, women don't have more severe cases than men who also have it. You're also at greater risk between the ages of 40-50 years old.

However, people of all ages have been diagnosed with CFS, including children. But children who develop the syndrome seem to have an easier time of it and it tends to go away faster.

Teenagers can come down with a case of glandular fever or 'kissing disease' as it's commonly nicknamed, that if left untreated is known to trigger lingering CFS.

There's also a connection between stress and chronic fatigue syndrome. It's thought that stress may trigger people who have a genetic predisposition for CFS to develop symptoms.

Alternatively, in our experience we have found that people who are overly stressed and who are already tired and run down and who then have a significant event happen in their life, especially an event that involves the use of antibiotics, are very likely to develop CFS.

This is such a common theme with the people we have spoken to that we believe there is a definite tie in with antibiotics as a trigger of this condition.

We find that up to half the people who we come in contact with who have CFS can identify conditions something similar to this in the 12 months prior to the onset of their condition.

Fear is the Enemy

Many people put off going to the doctor because they fear their possible diagnosis. But diagnosis is the first step toward wellness. Even if you do find you have something serious, it's better to know what you have and develop a plan to deal with it than to ignore it while the symptoms only worsen.

According to a study done by the Centers for Disease Control only about half of people with CFS have seen their doctor about it. That's a staggering number of people who haven't even been properly diagnosed.

You may be thinking that since there is no recognized cure for chronic fatigue syndrome it isn't necessary to deal with it in the doctor's office. But this couldn't be further from the truth. First, it's important to talk to your doctor so that you can rule out other possibilities.

Second, while there is no recognized cure there certainly are many ways you can manage chronic fatigue syndrome and get your life back. But if you don't know what you're dealing with, you can't make a great plan of attack.

Preparing for Your Visit to the Doctor

The more information you can give your doctor about your symptoms and triggers of them, the better.

It's a good idea to keep a detailed journal writing down each day the symptoms you experience and their duration as well as severity. Also include the things or events that you think may also trigger special symptoms.

You'll want to make sure you can share with your doctor:

- When you began to first notice your symptoms
- If anything makes symptoms worse or better
- Details of each symptom
- How your symptoms react to physical activity
- How your symptoms are at different times of the day

- Your current stress levels

You also need to provide a detailed medical history including:

- Medications you've taken or take now
- Surgeries you've had
- Illnesses you've had such viral infections or severe bacterial infections
- Family history of illnesses, especially fatigue
- Exposure to toxins
- Alcohol, drug, and tobacco use (past or present)
- Any other relevant health information

You should also write down any questions that you may have. Having a written list of things along with a journal of your symptoms is very valuable.

Be prepared to write down any notes from your discussions with the doctor during your visit as well. Don't rely on your memory in the hope that you will still remember it all when you get back home.

At Your Appointment

When you get to your doctor's appointment, make sure to bring along your journal and questions. When your doctor sees that you have come there fully prepared, you'll likely get more focused attention them.

Your doctor will likely ask you about your symptoms and then perform a physical exam. You should also expect that he or she will order blood tests to rule out other possible causes of your symptoms.

Some blood tests that may be performed include:

- CBC – complete blood count of white and red cells
- Thyroid level tests
- Liver function tests
- Blood sugar
- Creatine kinase
- Gluten sensitivity
- Urea
- Electrolytes

You may also be asked to provide a urine sample to check for proteins, sugar, white blood cells, and blood.

If any of the tests you're prescribed come back abnormal, you may be asked to take more tests to confirm a diagnosis or get more specific about it. Usually you'll schedule a second appointment to go over any lab results.

You should also ask for a copy of your lab results to keep for your own records. Having all of your health information together can help you if you need to go to see a specialist or have future health problems.

If all other tests come back normal and other possible causes of your health condition are ruled out, you may then be diagnosed with chronic fatigue syndrome.

The diagnosis isn't as cut and dry as we would like it to be, but in general you'll be diagnosed if:

- Other conditions are ruled out

- You have felt fatigue for at least one month and it isn't the result of exertion

- You have at least four of the most common chronic fatigue syndrome symptoms that have lasted for at least 6 months and have no other known cause

After you've been diagnosed, you'll be ready to take the next steps. This includes developing a plan to manage your chronic fatigue syndrome.

In the next three chapters we'll talk about different aspects of treatment that can help you to get your life back.

Does Your Doctor Understand and Treat Chronic Fatigue Syndrome?

Before we go too much further, though, it's important to discuss the type of doctor that you want to have on your team. Doctors are generally well educated and very good at what they do, but not all doctors are experts on CFS or really know how to treat it.

Some doctors may still be under the false idea that this is "all in your head" and you need to stay away from any doctor that doesn't see your illness as a true medical condition.

It's always a good idea to get a second opinion when you get a major diagnosis. A good doctor will be happy that you want to take this step and not feel threatened by it at all.

If you feel like your doctor isn't listening to you or is dismissing your symptoms, it's time to look for a new Doctor to treat you. But even if you have a caring and compassionate doctor, you may still need to find someone new if he or she doesn't really know how to help you manage your illness.

Unfortunately, there's no one specialty that is dedicated to the study of CFS. When you have cancer you go to an oncologist, when you have heart disease you see a cardiologist, but when you have CFS who do you see?

There are many ways you can go about looking for a physician that will be a good fit. Often you can get good treatment from a primary care or family medicine doctor if they've taken the time to become trained in this field.

If you need help finding a doctor who is able to really help you, there are several great methods for finding one referrals including:

- Talking to people in local CFS support groups and asking for referrals

- Referrals from people who practice complementary medicine such as chiropractors, massage therapists, and physical therapists

- Asking friends and family for a referral

- Talking with the staff of the doctor's office to find out if he or she has experience with CFS

- Making an appointment with a doctor and discuss his or her background with CFS

- Ask for a referral from your medical insurance company

When you meet with a doctor, the following are some good starter questions for your interview:

How many patients have you treated with CFS?

- What's your typical course of treatment for someone with this syndrome?

- Are you willing to research and/or participate in training on the latest treatment for CFS?
- How do you feel about complementary medicine such as massage therapy, acupuncture, herbal remedies, etc.?
- What lifestyle changes would you recommend for someone with CFS?

If your prospective doctor can answer these questions to your satisfaction and is open, friendly, and supportive then you have a good match. In the end, you need to trust your instincts about whether or not this will be a good fit for you.

What you don't want is someone who dismisses you, thinks you have a psychological disorder, or doesn't want to take time to learn more about the best ways to treat CFS.

Lifestyle Changes that Can Improve CFS

Chronic fatigue syndrome is one of those things that is really hard to overcome. In fact, studies and tests have shown that many people suffering from it never get over it entirely.

It may be that what you require is to learn enough that you can develop a lifetime management plan to better cope with CFS.

The fact is that even though you may not be able to completely get rid of this disease and forget about it, the quality of your life will improve if you go through proper therapy.

Different things have been reported to be successful with this syndrome. Some patients have stated that 'cognitive behavioral therapy' has worked wonders for them, while others claim that 'pacing' has been best in their case.

Still other people have stated that they responded best to 'graded exercise' therapy.

There is also a large group of patients who use 'nutritional supplementation' to improve their immune system and increase their energy levels. We are definitely in that group and each of us personally use our daily herbal based nutritional supplementation to manage our CFS.

As we said, fortunately there are many things that can be done, and in this chapter we will talk to you about each one of those things separately. You'll be able to select the types of therapy that you feel are best for you and even better, create your own individual mix to combine them for best results.

If you do decide to combine them, then you have to make sure that you don't overdo it.

You don't want to be unable to enjoy your life fully due to the fact that it is totally centered on overcoming CFS to the exclusion of anything else in life. It's best to take it easy and try to enjoy the process toward your recovery as much as possible.

Even though right now it might not seem like any therapy could be enjoyable, we will provide you with specific techniques and clarify the things that you may do to make this journey as pleasant as you can.

Using them you'll be able to regain the quality of life you've always desired.

Pacing Therapy

People suffering from chronic fatigue syndrome have a tendency to often forget that they are mere humans and that they need to rest more often than most people.

Instead, what they do is on their "good days" when they have a more energy, they tend to do everything all at once, before the usual tiredness kicks in.

The problem with that is that it can often lead to one good, productive day and then a few days where you cannot do anything. Here's what it will look like:

Let's say you have a great day. You feel energized and happy.

You decide to take care of everything you need to get done today, so you go and do the shopping, you do the laundry, you pick up the kids from school, you go to a bookstore and get the books you've always wanted to read.

Then you go visit a few friends, you cook a huge dinner, and you do the ironing because you know that if you get this done before your disease takes over, you can at least think that you're proactive that day.

Then the next day you realize that you're too tired to even get out of bed! You try to rest and relax, but the relaxation does not really help, and you just feel extremely exhausted.

Then, in the early afternoon, you still haven't really gotten anything done all day. The evening comes and you don't even have the energy to make dinner.

Then the same thing happens the next day.

The whole day goes by again and nothing really gets done. Now, the thing is that this can go on for days and even weeks. That is why the concept of 'pacing' yourself is so important.

Pacing allows you to manage your body and your physical ability in a way that will help you to feel good and stay active over extended periods of time.

To put it simply, if you apply pacing in your life, you may not get a whole lot of things done each and every day, but at least you do get something done each day, because you will have some energy daily.

Pacing will reduce the amount of time you spend passively getting over your chronic tiredness. It will help you to be more consistently productive for long periods of time.

There are a few things you need to understand about pacing, for it to work for you properly, and we will talk about those things in this chapter.

1. Understanding your own body.

It is impossible to implement pacing into your life without first knowing what your body is capable of doing at this stage of your illness.

Comparing yourself to others is no use here. What you need to do is to take a good look at yourself at your current level of health and decide what you really can or can't do.

To help you, we've come up with a few questions you can answer, and hopefully these answers will make it easier to judge your physical ability:

- How much physical work can you get done in a day or at a specific time?
- How much mental work can you get done in a day or at a specific time?
- What types of physical activity are the hardest for you?
- What types of mental activity are the hardest for you?
- What types of physical activity are the easiest for you?
- What types of mental activity are the easiest for you?
- When during the day do you have the greatest amount of energy?
- How does your body react to exertion and what are the first symptoms you can observe that will signal that you have reached your limit?

These questions are nothing revolutionary, but if you answer them honestly and truthfully, and if you observe yourself for a certain amount of time to really understand how your body reacts in various situations, you will then be better able to assess and use your feelings, your sensations and your own predictions to pace yourself well.

2. Be short and sweet.

Another thing you need to remember about pacing is that instead of trying to do everything at once, you need to divide your day into short periods of activity.

In between those periods, you'll need to take breaks that should be at least 15 minutes long. Think of it in terms of "chunking" your bigger daily chores into smaller bites or steps throughout the day.

If you're just starting out using pacing, you should remember to keep your activity periods very short.

For instance, try to start with doing tasks that you can get done in 10 minutes of activity and follow it with 15 minutes of rest. Try to stick this plan for a few days.

Then, you should look at yourself and ask yourself how you feel as a result of your past few days effort and exertion.

If you feel good, and if everything seems to be okay, then it will be possible for you to extend the periods of activity to say 15 – 20 minutes at a time.

After you make your activity periods longer, try not to change them for a few days. After a few days, look back once again at how you felt before and how you presently feel.

If you're feeling okay, then again you can extend each of your activity periods, remembering that you should have at least 15 minutes of rest in between each activity. During those breaks you can lay down on the floor or take a short nap.

Repeat the process of making the activity periods longer every few days until you don't feel comfortable with their length.

If you feel they are too long, and you become too tired as a result, just work backwards on the duration times to make them as short as you need until you feel comfortable again after completing your tasks.

When you find out what's best for you, stick to it and don't change it for some time.

Learning how to live and work around these much shorter activity periods may be a little stressful for you at times in the beginning, because it may be tempting for you to just keep working instead of taking a break.

It may be that after 30 minutes of work, you'll feel great and you want to keep going for a while longer, and then that becomes a little bit longer again… until!

Remember, despite the fact you may feel you have more energy during the actual activity period, you really do need to take that short break.

You need to remind yourself, that if you don't take a break now, you will have to deal with the consequences later on or the next day, and feeling regret later on will not undo the damage done.

3. Schedule your rest times.

Scheduling in general is a hard thing to do for most people. Especially, when you don't know how much time you actually have at your disposal to get tasks done before you get tired, or how energetic you will or will not feel on any given day.

It is tempting to create a very activity filled schedule for yourself on "good days" when you feel great, only to have the schedule totally unravel on the "bad days" when you experience low energy, and can't get through your tasks.

Even though you may know your body pretty well and think you know when you can expect to have a lot of energy and what times there is not going to be much to spare, your body will change constantly with this illness, and it will never be 100% predictable.

Here are a few tips that will make it easier for you to maintain and manage your relaxation and rest times during each day's schedule without feeling guilty:

Good rest is also time well spent.

You don't have to feel sorry or guilty for wanting to take a break. Everyone needs to rest, and when you suffer from CFS, it may be even more necessary to rest more frequently.

Resting will help you pace yourself.

There is a reason why I'm talking about scheduling rest in this chapter. If you do take the time to plan when you are going to take a break, you will end up taking care of yourself better, and you will have a lot more energy for the activities you really enjoy doing.

Be disciplined.

When you do decide to take a break at a set time, then you should be disciplined enough to actually carry out your plan and take that break.

Of course, it may be necessary for you to be flexible, just like we mentioned in the previous chapters, but unless something really extraordinary happenings that really requires your flexibility, you should stick to your plans as much as possible.

Understand how much rest you need.

Not everyone needs to take rest breaks in the same way. Some people with chronic fatigue syndrome require short frequent rests scattered through the day every 15-30 minutes, and others are okay with just 15 minutes of sleep every two hours.

You really need to find out what your body needs specifically, and provide it, so that your rest is as effective and as efficient as possible.

Again, there is no use in you comparing yourself to anyone else. The fact is that everyone is different, and because of that we need different things to function properly.

Then you can celebrate the milestones as you discover you need shorter or less frequent rest breaks.

But test it and adjust it at your own pace, don't be influenced by anyone else making demands on your time or having unrealistic expectations of what they think you should be able to do every day.

Learn to manage chaos.

When you first start scheduling your rest times, you'll realize that there are a lot of things going on, and it may be really hard for you to rest. Maybe your children will need some help, maybe your partner will need your opinion about something, maybe your friend will want to ask you how she looks in her new dress.

You want to be as nice to the people around you as possible, but by the same token you need to make sure that they understand that when you have a break, they really should not interrupt you unless they have something that absolutely cannot wait and has to be taken care of right away.

Remember that you can always ask your friends for assistance. Small children, disability or other personal circumstances may make it hard for you to plan effectively, but if you really try, and really put your heart to it, you will succeed.

There is absolutely no reason why you shouldn't be successful.

Hopefully the tips shared with you in this section will help you not only to plan well when you're going to rest but also will help you to understand how important it is to give up some of the non-essentials of what you think you absolutely have to do and take some time off in order for you to be able to function better for longer periods of time.

4. Have predictable and consistent routines.

Now we need to cover the need for you to establish stable routines in your life that you can rely on to remain consistent even in times of chaos.

You may be the type of person that does not like to plan everything, but if you are suffering from chronic fatigue syndrome, you will have to change your existing ways of doing things, or you will simply end up with more of the same that you already experience.

You will have to plan your days in such a way so that you don't end up going shopping, doing the laundry, working in the garden, etc. all on one single day. Instead, plan your laundry day on Tuesday, your garden day on Thursday, your shopping day on Monday, and so on.

Write up some realistic weekly timetables of what is pretty much guaranteed that you can get done even on a 'bad day' spread over the week's days.

This way you will do something every day, which will not only make you feel productive and efficient, but it will also help you to maintain a healthy balance in your life which is so needed when you have CFS.

Establishing routines will require cooperation from your entire family. You will need to tell them what you're planning to accomplish, so that they work with you and help you out as much as possible.

If you don't talk to them, the situation at your house may get really hectic.

Imagine that you are trying to set Friday as your day to do the shopping, but your husband does not realize that, and he eats all of your food by Wednesday.

Now, you have two choices, you can either go shopping on Wednesday, or you can wait until Friday, and stick to your original plan.

Of course another option that you have is sending your husband to do the shopping, but for the sake of this example, we will consider this option not available.

If you go shopping on Wednesday, then chances are you will overwork yourself and you will be really tired, maybe even too tired out to do anything on your schedule for Thursday, Friday, Saturday and Sunday.

If you have a feeling that is what is going to happen, obviously it is better for you make a decision to change your meal plans, or order out, or do send someone to get some emergency supplies, but stick to your own schedule to do your shopping normally as you planned on Friday.

At first you might have to stock up on a few extra things in your pantry so that you make sure that you don't run out of stores, but then you will just be able to do everything as scheduled, and you will learn how much to buy at each shopping trip, and not need to change that schedule.

Now, if you talk to your family beforehand, chances are it would not cause any trouble for them to make sure that there is enough food in the fridge until Friday. Who knows, maybe it would help them to be more thoughtful about what they eat and when, to help you not to have to deal with the stress of running out mid-week.

All you have to do is tell them about your plans.

The most important thing you need to remember about establishing consistent and achievable daily and weekly routines is that you shouldn't have more than one difficult or complicated tasks set out for the same day.

You should look at what you have to do during the week and plan it out in a way that you don't overwork yourself and don't get too tired.

Do the same for chores and activities that need to be done on a monthly or longer schedule basis, like the car wash, lawn mowing, spring cleaning, kid's trips and special events and so on.

Try to set it up so that if there is a difficult thing to do on Monday, make sure to plan for the rest of the things to do that day are all easy for you to complete.

Then again to set up one difficult thing for Tuesday and make sure that the rest of the things are again easy for you.

Do the same with Wednesday, Thursday, Friday, Saturday and Sunday.

Once your schedule is tested and proven to be an achievable schedule, and once your routines are established with suitable rest periods built into it, you really shouldn't need to change them unless there is a valid reason to.

If you stick to them for a few weeks and months, your body will get used to the labor required and adjust to the demands made on your body without experiencing undue stress, just like it gets used to working out every day when it is a well planned exercise routine custom made for you.

After some time, performing the same activities on the same days will be very easy for you and you will not get too tired.

The very last thing we want to talk to you about before the next chapter is making sure you understand that everything is manageable and everything can be scheduled.

Apply this system to your workplace activities as well if possible. Discuss your health problems with your supervisor and see if you can test new schedules that still allow for consistent activities to be achieved, evenly spread over the week, and with suitable rest periods allowed for.

At the very least, discussing your illness and explaining the pacing therapy with a Supervisor or HR manager will help you to implement your therapy steps without being judged unfairly for not being able to work at the level you used to.

You may find that your employer would prefer for you to try and work on even a slightly restricted basis, rather than risk losing you altogether from your untreated illness.

Obviously, if it happens that you have a situation that requires you to make an adjustment of the plan, then by all means go ahead and adjust it.

Establishing routines is extremely important for fighting CFS. It will be easier and easier the more you do it, so the hardest thing now is to just start doing it.

Diet & Nutrition for Beating CFS

There are two elements to diet and nutrition that you need to be aware of. The first is healthy eating and the second is dealing with the effects diet can have on your health and your day by day lifestyle (We will treat nutritional supplements as a separate subject).

1. Healthy Eating

Everyone knows that you should eat a balanced and healthy diet, which is generally a good thing, but it's especially important when it comes to CFS treatment.

The thing is that when you suffer from CFS, you are really tired all the time and to get rid of that feeling of constant fatigue, you need to eat as well as you possibly can with the best possible nutrition to help your new cells improve for your recovery on a cellular level.

In order to be able to have a balanced diet, you need to make sure you don't exclude any of your food groups.

The five food groups you should be especially concerned with are:

1. **Vegetables**
2. **Protein**
3. **Grains**
4. **Fruits**
5. **Dairy**

- To this you should add a focus of having adequate water in your diet

Some people claim that you should exclude some of the above groups when you're on a diet or in various other circumstances. Unless you have medical advice to the contrary then no matter what the situation is, you should always eat something from every one of those groups.

As a general guide, whole foods are best and the less processed your food is, the better. That means raw fruit and vegetables will be better than steamed ones. Steamed ones would be better than baked and processed vegetables and anything will be better than pre-packed, frozen then reheated vegetables. Not to mention fried vegetables!

A small serve of steak is a good protein source. But a commercial beef hamburger made with a premade beef patty that has been created somewhere else, frozen and shipped to the store and is served with a scattering of salad vegetables with a commercial sauce in a high sugar roll has such little nutrition or protein in it that it is difficult to even rate it as being food.

Fast food may taste good, and be a part of your social events, but do not confuse that with healthy eating. Taking time to eat a balanced and nutritious diet is one of the most basic and essential steps you can take towards improving your health.

You may not realize that when you suffer from Chronic Fatigue Syndrome, there are also certain foods that may be especially harmful to you.

If you have not done so already you should put some attention into understanding your personal food sensitivities. It is quite common for people with serious health issues, including people with CFS, to have food sensitivities and food allergies.

This may be Lactose Intolerance creating health challenges with milk products.

It may be Celiac Disease that gives you difficulty with gluten - making wheat, rye, barley and oats problematic in your diet.

Many people find chemicals in food: colorings and preservatives for example, give them adverse reactions.

We are not going to go into these things in depth here, but they are areas where you should pay attention. It's best to get some professional advice from your doctor, from a nutritionist, from a naturopath or from a food specialist.

We are in the process of writing a companion volume 2 to this book looking at detailed action steps you can take to work with CFS. In that volume we will devote a number of chapters to this. But for now we want to guide you on coming to grips with the problem and where and how to go and get advice in your local area

We are pretty much all aware of foods that are generally not good for people, so if a certain product does not seem to be good to eat generally, chances are you shouldn't eat it when you suffer from CFS.

Some examples of foods that may not be good for you include:

- high calorie foods
- deep fried foods
- refined sugar

Other things that are best for many CFS sufferers to avoid eating regularly or eating in quantity are:

- coffee
- sweets and candy
- alcohol products

This can be very difficult when you are at a low energy level, as most people will instinctively crave sugars, salts, caffeine and fats for a quick 'energy boost'.

You might be tempted to stop on the way to work in the morning for a cup of coffee with sugar, a donut, and or a packet of crisps. We have certainly done that in the past!

While it may work to make you feel better for a few minutes, the same ingredients quickly cause your levels to sink even lower than they originally were, and even make some people sleepy, within a very short time of eating them.

We have an important tip for you regarding caffeine: as you probably know, it stimulates people and makes it harder for them to sleep. The purpose of caffeine is to "wake you up in the morning", right?

The thing is that you probably have sleeping problems anyway, if you suffer from CFS. You shouldn't make it even harder for you to fall asleep, so you should really avoid things that will make it hard for you to fall asleep.

You should pay particular attention to how your body reacts to certain foods or drinks (such as energy drinks, carbonated drinks, etc) and see how you sleep after eating or drinking those things. If you think you can't start the day without caffeine, a tip you can benefit from is that the drink that wakes you up best is actually apple juice!

Again, we want to make sure that you understand that it is really all about self-observation and knowing how your body reacts to certain situations and foods.

What to do if you notice bad reactions to some foods

You should, as we said, get tested for possible food allergies, as you will need to eliminate those foods from your diet to take the stress off your already overwhelmed immune system.

And be aware of the effects food have on you when you eat. If you notice you feel more vitality from some foods than others, then increase them in your daily food plan.

Alternatively, if you notice that some foods decrease your energy levels, like some common carbohydrates sometimes do, then cut back on them.

If you feel extra sleepy after eating a bread sandwich or a donut or wheat crackers, then you need to be aware that those foods should be monitored and maybe not eaten during the working day time.

If any foods bring out an unusual reaction on your skin like hives or a rash, or your tongue / throat / gums start to feel swollen or sore after eating certain foods, or you experience stomach or bowel problems, then get tested for food allergies.

It's always best to begin with a healthy diet that's naturally full of vitamins and minerals. But adding healthy supplements can be a natural way to relieve the fatigue, pain, and mood problems that go along with chronic fatigue syndrome.

Nutritional Supplementation

There is a massive range of nutritional supplementation products available on the market. If you do a search of the internet for supplements that come with claims that they will help CFS, then you will find too many to count.

There will be so many being touted online, that trying to find what nutritional supplements are best for you could confuse you to the point of paralysis.

Some of these products will work for some people; others will be little or no use whatsoever.

In our experience the products that start out sounding like they could be useful for treating Chronic Fatigue usually end up actually being of little or no benefit for sufferers.

The problem here, in our opinion, is that the products that could be really useful in balancing your health end up doing very little to help because your body is unable to fully absorb the nutrition when you take it.

You may take a supplement, but since your body is unable to completely absorb the nutrition it just passes through the body and ends up in the toilet.

The key to using nutrition to assist with CFS is to begin the process by rebuilding the body's capacity to absorb the nutrition you are taking.

Herbal Based Nutritional Supplementation Products

We have been working for around 20 years with one range of natural herbal based nutritional supplementation products manufactured by the Herbalife company. They are best known in the marketplace for their weight control programs, in fact they are the world leader in that field.

These supplements focus on cellular nutrition. This means giving the body nutrition that is in total balance and that gives the body what it needs to nourish it on a cellular level. When you give the body the tools it needs it will often heal itself.

The thing that separates Herbalife products from anything else of the market is that the concept of cellular regeneration underpins these products. This allows your body to better rebuild your digestive process and you are better able to absorb the nutrition that the supplement products provide.

Both of the authors of this book, Helene and Warren, have had excellent personal results from using Herbalife products and they have turned out to be a key answer for our own CFS conditions.

Obviously that makes us a little biased in leaning towards supplements manufactured by Herbalife as being the best answer for nutritional supplementation therapy when working with CFS.

As part of the companion volume 2 we are adding a complete section with step by step guides on how to use nutrition products and what to expect when you do. It will have a section focusing exclusively on applying the principals and products of Nutritional Therapy in treating CFS.

We won't be going into too much detail here, but If you do want specific suggestions right now on generic nutrition supplementation products, then we have added contact details at the end of the book. Please feel free to contact us directly to ask any questions or to check on the availability of the companion volume 2.

For a lot of people the information on diet, rest, exercise and other therapies outlined in this book will be enough for your recovery when you implement them.

Ensuring you feed your body the best nutrition from all the food groups is common sense to support your body in its daily cellular regeneration and building of its immune system.

Specific Nutrition Products – Working with Herbalife products

In this volume we will just give a quick summary of what you might anticipate from including Herbalife products in your daily nutrition plan. This is one of the range of options that is open to you as you combat CFS in your own life.

If your situation is identified as being based on malabsorption of nutrition, then you would realistically expect to see some improvement in your symptoms within a week or two and steady improvement back to a normal life.

If your problem developed from exposure to a viral infection then the recovery process is generally a little more dramatic with good days where you feel fantastic, and bad days when you think that it is just not going to work for you.

The outcome we normally expect in those cases though is that the 'good days' get better and the 'bad days' are not as bad as they used to be. In time the day comes when you realize that on the bad days you are actually better and fitter than you used to be on your good days.

That is the time when you realize that you really are feeling better and what you will actually get your life back under your own control. This process generally takes 30 to 60 days before you really feel you are making solid progress and it is all working for you.

The third group we have worked with are people who had issues with chemical contamination.

Getting through that requires detoxifying the chemicals out of your system. Normally this means that people who are dealing with this problem through nutritional therapy often feel worse before they get better.

People going through this can take 30 to 60 days before they begin to see those 'good days' occurring regularly. Chemical problems underpinning CFS can commonly take 6 to 12 months before you really feel you have control of your life again and live normally and are not having to worry about the food you eat and the environment you are going into.

If you are looking for more details on how to use Herbalife products then check information online at this address: http://www.thehealthsuccesssite.com/Chronic-fatigue-syndrome.html. Through that page you will find a contact form which you can use to contact us directly with any questions you may have about using nutritional supplementation as a therapy for your CFS.

Other Fundamental Nutrition Requirements

Vitamin C

You have to make sure that your diet does contain all of the necessary vitamins to help your body rebuild a strong immune system. Vitamins are important for your immune system to work properly which will cause you to be less tired as well as being able to be more productive.

One of the most important vitamins that you have to pay particularly close attention to is vitamin C. Vitamin C helps when your collagen gets formed, which in turn gives structure to your bones and even muscles or blood vessels.

It also helps to absorb iron and may prevent the common cold, which obviously can be a cause of why you won't be able to get very many things accomplished. On top of your regulars CFS symptoms, the common cold will add on to your tiredness and fatigue.

This vitamin cannot be created by the body itself and needs to be taken in from outside nutritional sources. That is why you need to take it in as food or drink or you can buy supplements that will help you to supply your body with this necessary vitamin.

There are many fruits and vegetables that are a great source of vitamin C. Those include strawberries, olives, kiwifruit, mango, broccoli and even very many juices that contain vitamin C.

If you like the leafy vegetables or fresh tomatoes, Brussels sprouts or broccoli, you will be able to get enough vitamin C quickly.

Vitamin E

Another vitamin that is crucial for you is vitamin E which is a very well-known antioxidant.

It works to help neutralize the free radicals in your body, which will have a twofold effect on you. One, it may make you look younger and two, it may help to strengthen your immune system dramatically.

It is recommended for both men and women to take vitamin E every day. Men should consume about 10 mg of it every day, and women should make sure to take in at least 8 mg a day.

Again, as was the case with vitamin C, there are many natural sources of vitamin E.

If you like avocado, whole grain bread, margarine and even vegetable oil, or nuts, and if you like liver you'll most likely be taking in as much of vitamin E as you require.

Zinc

What zinc does is to increase the number of cells that will kill diseases and infections quickly. If you combine it with vitamin C, you will be helping out your immune system and your body to fight disease.

It naturally strengthens your immune system because it helps your body to produce enough cells to heal from attacks.

Zinc may help you to deal with conditions such as the common cold, diabetes, arthritis, PMS, regeneration of your muscles, the flu, and of course the chronic fatigue syndrome.

If you want to take in enough zinc for you to function properly, you should eat summer squash, shrimp, peas, yogurt, maple syrup, lamb and beef, as well as sesame seeds and pumpkin seeds.

So, these are the three major nutritional supplements that you absolutely have to make sure you do include in your diet, whether in tablet form or from foods.

Of course it's ideal when you can take them naturally in fruits and vegetables, but if you don't have access to any of the fruits and vegetables that we have talked about above, then buying diet supplements that are of high quality will help immensely.

Generally speaking avoid all harmful foods or drinks that will make you feel worse, at the same time remembering what particular foods and drinks make you feel better.

There are several other antioxidant supplements that are good to try for improving your energy, mental health, and overall wellness including:

- Colloidal Silver – considered an immune booster that may relieve some CFS symptoms
- Omega 3 Fish Oil – these are heart healthy, but can also improve the connections in your brain and help to improve your mood
- Olive Leaf Extracts – have similar properties of fish oil
- Echinacea – a natural antibiotic that may also help boost your immunity and relieve CFS

Experiment with your nutrition and your supplements. Keep them natural and not artificial foods or artificially created supplements.

Learn what foods give you energy, and which ones leave you feeling drained and listless. Discover whether the 'lift' you feel from certain food is an artificial and short-term boost in energy, from a deceptive source like a sugar lift, or if the food gave you a sustainable energy increase that you still enjoy hours after eating it.

The more you listen to your body and the more you choose to eat natural and unprocessed foods, the more likely you are to support your other therapies for a sustainable reduction in your symptoms.

In volume 2 of this series of CFS Therapy books we will explore all the avenues and therapies as well as the specific herbal based nutritional products that we know have had exceptional benefits to our own health and for the people we have also assisted to better manage their CFS.

Exercise

When you have chronic fatigue, the last thing you probably want to do is to exercise. But exercise can be very beneficial in support ing your wellness. It is a therapy strategy that can help to make your immune system, muscle, bones, lungs, and mind stronger.

But when you have chronic fatigue syndrome, you need to approach exercise differently than if you were trying to get a 'beach body'. Starting out slowly and being consistent in your efforts is the key to success.

The principles of pacing are important to remember here. Begin with just five minutes of an exercise routine. Something as simple as taking a short stroll down the street, or wandering around your home garden, may work just fine for your program when you first start out.

Consistently exercises (or just 'move more' than usual) for five minutes at a time for a week or two. Then, when you feel a little stronger you can add to your routine and add a few minutes to the routine.

Continue to do this until you can manage 30 minutes of activity daily – and don't worry if that takes you many weeks to achieve.

You may be tempted to do more on "good days" when you have high energy. But it's not a good idea to overdo it on high energy days.

Be consistent whether you have high or low energy when you exercise. Stick to the schedules and daily workout routines that you have set for yourself. And be sure to stick also to your Rest schedules to allow suitable recovery time after each exertion of effort.

Over time you'll begin to feel the benefits of this increased activity every day. You'll feel stronger and you'll notice an increase in the amount of available energy you have. If weight loss is something you need, this will also help you to maintain a healthier weight.

Exercise also helps you to have improved mental health. In fact, studies have shown that exercise can be as effective as antidepressants in helping to improve your mood. Something that's very beneficial when you're dealing with CFS.

What kinds of activities are good for people with CFS? You may be bored with only walking, though it's a great exercise. Here are some other options that may be good for you:

- yoga
- stretching
- swimming or water aerobics
- bicycling
- Pilates

These exercises are gentle on the body and can help improve both your body and mind as you add them to your lifestyle. Variety can be a very good way to stay committed to exercise, just make sure you stay consistent with the amount of energy you expend.

Detoxification

One of the risk factors for chronic fatigue syndrome is exposure to toxins. And toxins are all around us. They can be in the food you eat, the air you breathe, and on just about any surface you touch.

It's often helpful to follow a detoxification protocol in order to rid your body of toxins and get relief from your chronic fatigue syndrome symptoms. There are several ways you can do this.

First, begin with your diet. As we've already discussed sugar can be a major problem that exacerbates CFS. Eliminating sugar from your diet will naturally help you to detoxify.

You can also find nutritional supplements specifically designed to help you detoxify the liver, gall bladder, and your bowels. Usually these are a series of supplements that you take daily over a period of several days.

You may also be instructed to undertake what is called a Fast for the time period when you follow the supplements, by eliminating certain foods and drinking plenty of fluids. These are generally safe for short periods of time and can help your body to remove many of the toxins that have built up in it.

Massage can also help to move the lymph fluid around in your body and to detoxify your muscles and the tissues below the skin. Deep tissue massage is the most effective at doing this.

You may also talk with your chiropractor or a doctor of osteopathic medicine to perform a lymph cleansing procedure. This is a procedure that helps to loosen and move lymph fluid and get it pumping properly so that you can have better toxin removal.

Using the popular "Far Infrared Saunas" is also a great way to remove toxins. Saunas often help you to sweat out the toxins, but it can be difficult for someone with CFS to tolerate long bouts of heat.

With the Far Infrared Saunas you'll get detoxification without having to spend a long time in the heat. After you sauna, it's important to then shower so that the toxins are literally washed away.

Detoxing the Mind and Spirit

It's just as important to get rid of the toxic thoughts and negativity that can draw negative energy toward you.

Get a copy of a good quality 'Law of Attraction' book, or study something like 'The Secret' or 'What the Bleep do we Know'

DVD, to learn about the benefits of positive thinking and how to use positive energy for your health.

You do get, or attract to yourself, more of what you think about and focus on the most, so make it as positive and beneficial as possible. You may be surprised by how much negativity you are bringing into your beliefs about your therapy and your expectations of a recovery from CFS!

Practicing meditation, guided imagery, and working to stay away from negative influences can be as beneficial as some of the physical treatments.

That may mean avoiding media that represents violence and negativity. Be fussy about what you watch on TV and what movies you will give your attention to. Find shows and movies that make you laugh out loud!

Try only reading the weekly Sunday newspapers as they allocate more space to the 'good news' stories of the week instead of only presenting the daily disasters.

It may also mean avoiding any toxic people in your life and workplace who never seem to have anything nice to do or say. They drain your energy just listening to them and being in the same room.

You feel depressed and stressed when they demand your attention. Some toxic people enjoy creating anxiety and drama at every opportunity, constantly causing fights and uncomfortable scenes about unimportant matters.

If you groan inside at the thought of spending time with someone, or your jaw clenches and stomach sinks, then listen to what your body is telling you about the effect this toxic person has on your overall well-being. These are signals to avoid being around them if you can.

On the other hand, spending more time with positive people can be very healing. You may be lucky enough to know someone who can brighten any day, and that makes you feel good about yourself when you are in their company.

If you don't – then go looking to find someone like that! They may be already in your family or social circle, but you haven't yet made a project out of finding and recognizing them as the treasure they are to your well-being.

You can also work to look for the good already being experienced in your everyday life. Keeping a "gratitude journal" can help you to identify and dwell on the good things that are happening each day and focus your energy on them.

Remind yourself every day of the things and events that make you happy, feel abundant, the things that you would like to experience more of. Be grateful for what you have and be optimistic about being able to have and attract even more of these things and events.

Focusing on having a positive attitude will help you to heal. If you believe that you can beat chronic fatigue syndrome, then you will.

But if you spend all of your time worrying or with self-defeating thoughts about never getting better, or how hard it is to cope with the way you feel now, you will have a harder time beating the syndrome.

Remember that the mind and body are intimately connected and when you improve one of them, the other follows. Using the power of your mind to heal and feel well is very powerful.

Probiotics

Antibiotics are so overprescribed that we often don't have enough healthy bacteria in our bodies. Much of our food supply is also tainted with antibiotics used in commercial agriculture.

But there are many species of bacteria that are healthy for the body and that we need in order to have strong immunity and good digestion to get rid of toxins. There are a few different ways you can improve the bacteria levels in your body.

First, you can take nutritional supplements. There are acidophilus supplements that contain one type of bacteria. There are also supplements specifically made with a wider variety of bacteria.

You can also eat food that's enriched with probiotics such as natural yogurt and kefir. These help to naturally boost your bacteria levels. Also, avoid foods that have been processed using antibiotics.

Look for labels on dairy and meat products that specifically say "antibiotic free". Organic products that are certified are also free from this treatment that can make its way into your system.

Keep Candida in Check

Candida is a type of yeast that naturally occurs in the healthy body – and all around us. We need to have some of it in the body so that things stay in natural balance.

But when you kill off too much bacteria in the body or take in too much sugar, yeast can become overgrown.

We typically think of yeast infections being a problem that women deal with in their reproductive system. But yeast can actually take over the entire body and cause chronic problems with fatigue.

You can help to eliminate candida by avoiding foods that have yeast in them such as breads and other leavened foods. You can also eliminate sugar which feeds the yeast.

Learn more about the nutritional therapies that help to fight yeast and build your strength. Finally, adding probiotics will help to keep yeast from becoming overgrown.

The Restorative Power of Sleep

One of the hallmarks of chronic fatigue syndrome is that you're unable to get refreshed from your nightly sleep. In addition, even though you feel exhausted, you may find that getting to sleep in the first place is almost impossible.

We talked before about the need for scheduled rest and protecting your energy levels. Now we want to look in more depth at this and give you some tools to get the sleep you need.

You might develop very irregular sleep patterns that make you feel even more miserable. It's important to try to develop a consistent sleep pattern regardless of what might come naturally to you with CFS.

Some helpful tips to improve your sleep:

- Go to bed at the same time each night, even if you don't feel like it
- Wake at the same time each day even if you don't feel like it
- Make sure you schedule 8-10 hours of sleep each day
- Keep distractions such as television to a minimum in your bedroom, and don't work on your laptop or do other work that requires to you wake up and concentrate on it

- Make your bedroom a peaceful environment – comfortable bedding, supportive mattress, free from clutter or distractions
- Avoid caffeine and sugar at least 5 hours before bed
- Learn what foods and drinks are said to help improve sleep, and start testing some for yourself
- Try a natural supplement such as melatonin to help you establish a regular sleep routine
- Use white noise recordings to keep you from hearing sounds that might make it difficult to sleep
- Make sure your room is not too warm – cool rooms tend to be more conducive to sleep
- Use the least amount of bedding and blankets you can comfortably sleep with to keep your body temperature from becoming too hot in your sleep
- Create an environment of total darkness for sleep – you may have to black out windows and keep the amount of electrical gadgets that blink lights and have illuminated screens etc. to a minimum. Use a sleep mask if you have to
- In the evening, use as little artificial light as possible so that your body gets the signals to prepare for sleep

It may take some time, but eventually you'll begin to develop a pattern of sleep and rest that helps you to consistently have more energy. Even if you're not able to fall into a deep sleep, you'll at least get consistent rest.

Guard Your Energy Reserves

There are many things in life that threaten to steal your energy and leave you depleted.

It's important to make sure that you don't let anyone take it away from you if you don't have it to give. That could mean people in your life that are very demanding and consume your mental, emotional, and physical energy.

You love your friends and family, but you need to learn to say "No" when they expect or even demand, too much from you. Be guilt free when you have to say "No" to their requests.

It could be a stressful job that needs to change as soon as you can find something else. You may be surprised to find that your supervisor or employer is understanding about your illness and supportive of your pace therapy. If not, then you need to consider which is more important to your life long wellbeing.

It could also be that you have impossibly high standards for yourself. Often we are the ones who make life difficult for ourselves.

Some people take pride in being 'perfectionists' but that is only another way to put unrealistic expectations on your performance levels. Learn that sometimes 'good enough' really IS good enough.

Be kind to yourself and realize that you may not be able to do all that you did before the CFS came knocking on your door. Become realistic about what is achievable each day, and make allowances for the fact that you will have some 'bad days' that trip up even the best laid plans.

Be careful to prioritize what's most important and avoid taking on more than you can really handle. Work with the people in your life to get help with tasks that might drain you of energy, but still need to be done.

As soon as you begin to apply the pacing strategies and create realistic schedules around your life, you will begin to see how in the past you have not been guarding your energy reserves from being drained and even wasted.

Avoid Addictive Habits

Addiction by its very nature drains you of energy and resources. You become a slave to the things you're addicted to, be it alcohol, drugs, tobacco, or even behaviors such as gambling or shopping.

If you've managed to avoid these habits so far in life, don't start any of them now. Chances are if you make it into late adulthood without an addiction you won't begin one. However, the stress of dealing with chronic illness can drive you to look for something to fill the void.

It is tempting to think that something like alcohol or comfort foods can give you an energy boost, or simply make you 'feel better' than you do right now, but that would be totally wrong, and could lead to a seriously unhealthy addiction very quickly.

If you're already in the throes of an addiction, this is a good time to seek help. Some addictions may require professional help or support groups. This tends to be the case with alcohol, drugs, and other behavioral addictions.

Many find success in 12 step programs and there are programs for just about any addiction including:

- Alcoholics Anonymous
- Narcotics Anonymous
- Overeaters Anonymous
- Gamblers Anonymous

While we often think of smoking as being an easier habit to break, the truth is that it's a terribly addictive substance that's very difficult to stop using. There is often help from professionals available. Talk with your doctor about aids to stop smoking.

You may also want to look in your local community center, hospital, or clinic for a smoking cessation group that meets to help provide support. Once you kick the habit of smoking you'll feel better and you'll save a lot of your money.

No matter how long you've struggled with an addiction, there's hope for people who want to quit. But often you'll need help from others to do it, so don't be afraid to reach out for assistance.

Removing an addiction from your life will help to restore mental, physical, and spiritual balance to your life. It will draw more positive energy to you and help you to beat chronic fatigue syndrome as well.

Medical Treatment for Chronic Fatigue Syndrome

We've spent a lot of time discussing what you can do for yourself, but there are also some medical treatments that have been helpful in dealing with chronic fatigue syndrome symptoms.

In this chapter we'll include medical treatment as well as 'cognitive behavioral therapy' that are administered by a professional. Together you may find that these can help you to overcome CFS symptoms that can't be relieved through lifestyle changes alone.

There are no drugs specifically designated for chronic fatigue syndrome and there's no specifically prescribed medical cure for this illness. But physicians can prescribe drugs that help alleviate the symptoms and help you to cope.

Antidepressants

Antidepressants can provide you with some relief from CFS. Depression and any chronic disease go hand in hand, and having some help to improve your depression may help you to cope better with the changes you need to make in your lifestyle.

These medications also can work to help you sleep better and relieve pain because of the way they work with the neurotransmitters in the brain. It is not uncommon for very long-term CFS patients to become almost suicidal with depression and hopelessness about ever finding any way to recover.

If you ever feel that degree of depression that it is life-threatening, you must seek medical assistance. While these medications may not be needed long-term, they can help you to get through a flare up of CFS.

Anti-Inflammatories

With chronic fatigue syndrome you can have symptoms such as muscle pain and sore throat. Anti-inflammatories can help you to get some pain relief so that your daily activities are easier to perform.

Especially since CFS tends to work hand-in-hand with other severe chronic illnesses like rheumatoid arthritis, you may experience severe joint inflammation and pain at various times.

Make sure that you get tested for other illnesses that may be causing pain so that you have a complete pain management and anti-inflammation treatment plan in place.

You can get some anti-inflammatories over the counter and for some you are required to have a prescription. This is another treatment that can help you as you transition into new lifestyle behaviors that will provide long-term relief.

Sleeping Medication

If you're struggling to sleep at night, you may benefit from sleeping pills that can help you to fall asleep and stay asleep through the night. This can help you to establish a new pattern for sleep.

It's important to note, though, that sleep medications can become habit-forming. That means you may get to a point when you can't sleep without them. These are best used for short-term help while you're first testing and adjusting to your new lifestyle.

Developing your own most ideal sleep routine is the best way to ensure recuperative sleep. But by all means use whatever tools are available to you while you are testing and developing your best sleep hygiene.

Natural supplements such as melatonin may be beneficial and not habit-forming. You can also try natural sleep remedies such as taking a warm bath or drinking chamomile tea before bed.

CBT - Cognitive Behavioral Therapy

This is a general overview of what has become a popular therapy for CFS that your doctor may prescribe for you.

The whole purpose of 'cognitive behavioral therapy' in treating chronic fatigue syndrome is to help people regain control of their life.

What needs to happen is the patient needs to change the way they perceive and think about their tiredness and fatigue. After that change is made they can change their behavior accordingly.

Also, if cognitive behavioral therapy is successful, the patient will be able to manage his problems better, such as get rid of sleeping problems as well as improve stress management.

This type of therapy is usually performed over a number of sessions that a patient has to attend. Each session lasts for about an hour and there are from six to 20 sessions in the therapy.

As the therapy progresses, it may be necessary for CFS patients to have to do things that they used to avoid because of negative experiences in the past, such as going out for walks or playing sports.

There are several components to cognitive behavioral therapy. Let's take a look at a few of them.

Keeping a Journal

A CBT patient will be asked to keep a detailed journal which will become a guide for planning things to do and setting reasonable limits in life.

The patient will keep that journal and use it to track important things such as relationships, jobs, or other activities that may make them feel more tired or emotionally engaged.

They will also be asked to record the times during the day they feel more exhausted, and when they are relaxed and refreshed. This will help them to adjust their lives and their schedule so they can get the most out of their time.

Changing Your Schedule

As mentioned in the previous paragraph, a cognitive behavioral therapy patient will be asked to look over his schedule and adjust it according to his energy downfalls and peaks.

What this means is that patients have to determine when they have energy peaks and change their schedules so that they can use those peaks for the most important activities during the day.

This will then be used for developing the daily routines we discussed earlier here, which will improve the quality of their lives.

Changing Your Attitude

Most all the things that we go through in life happen in our heads. It is true that if we change the attitude towards something, we can change the most negative situations into positive and even pleasing ones.

Chronic fatigue syndrome patients have a tendency to think very little of themselves and suffer from low self esteem issues. They think they are not active enough and that they are not productive enough to be considered valuable contributors to family and

friends, as well as on the job. They also have a tendency to think that they cannot control their disease.

Cognitive behavioral therapy will attempt to change your thinking from negative to positive.

As a result, instead of focusing on being a failure, not being in control etc, you will focus on the instances where you managed to overcome the disease for at least a short amount of time.

Once you are able to pinpoint a few such instances, you will start thinking better of yourself and then your self-esteem will grow, and the quality of your life will improve.

Maintaining Flexibility

Although keeping a journal helps to decide when and how the energy levels will go up, the truth is that this is not simply a math problem to solve. People are not machines, and you're not working with a mechanism. This is your body we are talking about and your body is not a machine.

That is why your energy levels are not always going to be completely predictable. In some cases it will be difficult for you to know when you are going to have a productive time during the day.

That is why you have to be flexible enough to quickly react to energy level changes.

If you see, for example, that even though you are expecting to be out of energy during a specific time during the day, you feel energized and strong, be ready to change the schedule to take advantage of that energy boost.

Another technique is to take short naps frequently during the day and combine them with meditation as well as relaxation. This will help you to better notice and remain active during your energy peak.

Another thing that will be present doing cognitive behavioral therapy is breaking down complex things to do into small tasks and then managing them.

This will help the patients to set limits and make sure that they will not get discouraged or stressed out when trying to cope with a complicated situation.

The truth is that everyone gets stressed when they think that something is too formidable for them to deal with. Usually, people can manage that stress without much trouble, but chronic fatigue syndrome patients will have a really hard time with it.

That is why it is best for them to just take their tasks one step at a time and try to focus on one simple thing at a time. This is an important skill and CFS patients will learn it when in therapy.

Prioritizing

Of course it is important for everyone to prioritize, no matter if they do have chronic fatigue syndrome or not.

The problem is that if you are running out of energy all the time, you have to create your schedule around your priorities so that you're able to actually take care of them before you run out of strength.

That is why you have to plan your day out really well and you have to be able to decide which things are most important in which things can wait until the next day.

The worst thing that can happen is a patient putting too much on his shoulders and then getting discouraged and unmotivated.

That is why, during cognitive behavioral therapy, prioritizing is very strongly emphasized and a considerable amount of time is spent learning that important skill.

Learning to Focus

CFS patients participating in CBT will also learn how to concentrate. They will be taught how to increase their uptime through working on developing their alertness.

To put it simply, a patient will be taught to stay alert when he needs to so that he can function properly. That also means that he will be able to identify times when focusing is not needed and he can unwind and relax.

Dealing with Relapses

People get discouraged when they work on something but realize that they're not making much progress.

Imagine a situation where you're trying to quit smoking, but instead of just quitting and forgetting about it, you take out a cigarette a week after you decided not to smoke again and light it with great pleasure.

What do you think is going to happen after you smoke? You are going to think to yourself that you have just failed, and "this whole quit smoking thing" does not make sense anymore.

Possibly, you are even going to give up trying to quit smoking altogether. You should not ever quit trying even though it may take several failures for you to finally succeed.

If the first time you tried to accomplish something and you are not successful, just don't worry about it and try again next time. The time will come when you will be successful.

CFS patients also go through very similar struggles, but they are much more intense for them. An important part of cognitive behavioral therapy is teaching those patients how to accept difficulties as well as the fact that they may sometimes fail, and that they may have to start over sometimes.

As you have probably seen from this chapter, 'cognitive behavioral therapy' is focused around self-discipline and self-observation.

During the therapy patients change their way of thinking and looking at the world. If the therapy is successful, the world is not a negative place for them anymore. It's not a place where they are always tired and cannot really accomplish anything.

Instead, it becomes a very positive place where they can do anything they want, and even though it might be hard for them sometimes, they will be successful at leading a happy life.

You will have noted that many of the therapies covered in this book can also be seen represented in CBT, but are under your own control as a self-help therapy and treatment plan instead of being supervised by a doctor.

Why Does This Cognitive Behavioral Therapy Work?

The fact is that if you do something for long enough, it will become your nature. Remember that you must practice a new pattern, routine or behavior for at least 30 days before it begins to become an automatic and unconscious part of your behavior.

It may feel awkward and uncomfortable for the first month when you are learning and adapting your therapy plan.

Even though at first it may be difficult for cognitive behavioral therapy patients to change, after some time and practice the new and improved way of thinking becomes their second nature and they don't even have to think about it anymore. Becoming a positive thinker just comes to them naturally.

Even though this therapy may not cure CFS 100%, it may greatly improve the quality of your existence. You will need to contact a professional to help guide you through this process.

Talk with people in local chronic fatigue syndrome support groups to find a local professional who is experienced with this type of intensive therapy. You may also want to talk with your doctor about a recommendation.

Remember that CFS Is Not Like Other Health Conditions

Have you ever had the feeling when you went to the doctor that you hope they'll find something wrong with you? That way you can be 'treated' by them and on your way to being healthy again.

What can be frustrating with CFS is that being diagnosed doesn't equal treatment or a cure. Because the medical community has only recently begun studying this illness, or even acknowledging it, there aren't many medical options yet.

Once you're diagnosed with chronic fatigue syndrome you can be relieved that you don't have an illness that will end your life. But with this syndrome you'll be responsible for a lot of the changes that take place to improve your condition.

Many people find that medical treatment can initially help to control pain and depression while making the necessary lifestyle changes to have long-term wellness without medical intervention.

Seek Support When Trying Out Cognitive Behavioral Therapy

Remember that you're not alone and seeking support from others will be critical to your own recovery. Look for a local support group to help you learn tips and strategies for coping with this illness.

If you're not able to attend a local Cognitive Behavioral Therapy support group, you'll be able to find many online communities where people share their stories of both frustration and hope. Sometimes you just need to vent to people who personally understand what you're going through.

While many people that care about you can be supportive, there's something powerful about having relationships with people who are facing the same problems and developing greater understanding of the condition together.

Complementary Therapies to Manage CFS

While Western medicine can sometimes be disappointing with its limited offerings, you can look to complementary medicine to offer help for chronic fatigue syndrome. There are many options for you if you're willing to experiment with alternative medicine.

Chinese Medicine

Chinese medicine works with the body's energy systems to help restore balance. This ancient art sometimes has answers to the questions that Western medicine has yet to solve.

It's less concerned with finding a pathogen than it is with helping your body naturally be restored to a balanced state. If you go to a practitioner of Chinese medicine, there may be many therapies that can help you such as:

- Chinese herbs
- Acupuncture
- Cupping
- Moxibustion
- Massage

These treatments can be very effective at helping to relieve pain, reduce stress, improve your mood, and help you sleep. None of these therapies are painful and, in fact, can be quite relaxing and peaceful.

When you go to see a practitioner of Chinese medicine, your first appointment will be to get acquainted and to discuss the state of your health. Your practitioner will take a detailed history from you and then examine your tongue and take your pulse to make a diagnosis.

If you've never experienced it before, this process can feel a little strange. But it's worked for many thousands of years and many people report improvement after receiving treatment.

You'll want to look for a practitioner that has education and training in Chinese medicine and believes in its philosophy – not someone who went to a weekend workshop on acupuncture.

Ask about education, training, and professional certifications and licenses before making an appointment.

Massage Therapy

Massage can help to remove toxins from the body and bring comfort to sore muscles. This is a wonderful way to get relief from stress as well. You'll want to work with a massage therapist who is familiar with chronic fatigue syndrome and techniques that will aid in your healing.

It's becoming more and more common for doctors to understand the benefits of massage and prescribe it as a treatment for CFS. Talk to your doctor about this option as it can be paid for by health insurance in many instances.

Swedish massage is relaxing and will give benefits to you. But you're more likely to get the most powerful benefits from deep tissue massage. This isn't quite as relaxing and can even be uncomfortable at times, but it can help you to feel more energy.

Apart from anything else, massage is a wonderful way to get back in touch with your body, and to become more aware of your physicality. When you are ill for extended periods of time it becomes normal to feel that your body has betrayed you and you want to punish your body.

Massage helps you to deeply relax, and to enjoy the healing touch of the masseur, and to begin developing a more positive and loving relationship with your body once again.

Physical Therapy

Physical therapy is often helpful for people who need help with pain relief and to increase your physical activity. Graded exercise programs are often helpful for improving your wellness and energy levels.

Ask your doctor to refer you to a physical therapist to help you get started with a program to relieve your symptoms. Physical therapy requires hard work on your part to make progress, but it's worth it.

Energy Medicine

Energy medicine is the term for a broad category of treatments. But the basic idea is that energy flows through your body and when it's blocked or corrupted by negative energy, you have illness.

Practitioners of energy medicine use a wide variety of techniques to help you get energy flowing smoothly again and to remove negative energies that may be in the way of your healing.

Some examples of energy medicine include:

- Reiki
- Acupuncture
- Reflexology
- Distance healing
- Vibrational healing
- Kinesiology
- Prayer and meditation

Many people have felt comfort and healing by using these methods of healing.

If you're interested in them, look for a local professional to guide you through the process.

You can also get many books on self-healing through 'energy medicine' that can help you as well.

Chiropractic Care

Chiropractors can help you to have better alignment of your bones which helps your nervous system to function properly. This type of care can be very helpful in treating symptoms of chronic fatigue syndrome and helping you to experience healing.

Many chiropractors are also affiliated with massage therapists and acupuncturists who can help you get a well-rounded treatment for your symptoms.

Talk with your prospective chiropractor to find out what experience he or she has with CFS – you want to work with someone who understands your needs.

Homeopathy

You may want to consult a practitioner of homeopathic medicine to determine a course of treatment. This is someone who can prescribe herbs, creams, and other non-pharmaceutical therapies.

When it comes to CFS, Western medicine is terribly limited.

A homeopathic practitioner can give you treatment options that can help provide you with pain relief, help to stabilize your mood, and give you more energy.

Look for someone who has a doctorate in homeopathic medicine and is highly trained to prescribe natural remedies for your problems. You may also find that he or she prescribes dietary changes as well.

Aromatherapy

Your senses are heavily influenced by what you smell, and learning about the power of aromatic oils as well as the benefits of specific scented plants, may also help you in managing CFS.

There are many scents and oils that relax, calm and balance your mind and body, while others are known for being able to stimulate, refresh, and energize your senses. Test some of the oils, scented candles, bath oils or salts, and scented herb pillows that are on the market and collect the ones that resonate best with your needs.

For example, Helene is always using Eucalyptus oil as an air spray or in a water and oil burner during winter, as it is said to help reduce contact with cold bugs, while also refreshing the stuffy air in the heated house, and helps to energize and refresh your senses.

Dietitian

Finally, a dietitian can be a wonderful source of information for you. Food can often be used as a medical treatment for restoring your body's nutrition and balance.

Look for a registered dietitian who has worked with people who have CFS before.

Remember that he or she can give you suggestions, but it will be up to you to implement those suggestions. Again, you always need to be a partner in your own treatment program.

In volume 2 of this CFS Therapies book set we will discuss in great detail the various aspects of nutritional therapy for your recovery on a cellular level.

Rebounding from Relapses

As you test the various therapies to learn what's best for your own chronic fatigue syndrome treatment, you may go through periods of time when you feel that you're over it and are "cured".

For some very fortunate people, the symptoms of chronic fatigue syndrome do go after a few months, never to return.

But for many people a period of remission is followed by a relapse of the syndrome. This can be a devastating blow when you've worked so hard to get through the period of more acute illness you've experienced.

Be Aware of Your Cycles

Many people who have CFS find that it flares up in a cyclical fashion.

As Helene explains, "In my own experience I have a flare up where I feel acute symptoms for about a week. During this time I am exhausted, feel sick, have aches and pains and feel depressed.

But with consistent application of these CFS therapies I start to feel better and better over the following days.

And then about 90 days later after feeling better and having energy the cycle starts over again and I'm plunged back into the CFS symptoms for another week.

Just when I start to feel normal again I get struck down by the next relapse. And my experience isn't unusual. "

Many others experience these cycles that can last anywhere from 90 to 120 days.

Do you remember that we asked you to keep a journal of your symptoms? This is a good practice to continue so that you can find your own patterns and cycles.

While it never feels good to have a relapse, it can help you to know what might be coming in the days ahead and to prepare yourself.

Two Steps Forward, One Step Back

A relapse may make you feel that all the progress you made was for nothing. But it's not as bad as you might think. As you begin to experience healing from chronic fatigue syndrome, you really are getting better.

But there are bound to be setbacks along the way. These don't take away from all that you've learned about self-care and healing. You are still making progress; you just need to remember that it is a long process.

Triggers for Relapse

While you're working hard on strengthening your immune system, your body gets better and better at clearing out toxins and fighting foreign invaders.

And your cells are beginning to replicate themselves with healthier copies of their cells, to better fight invaders and build your immune system. But many things can trigger a relapse of your CFS symptoms.

Some examples of triggers are:

- Very stressful situations
- Contact with a virus, bacteria, or other pathogen
- Exposure to toxins
- Lack of self-care (in other words, neglecting the pacing and patterns you've used earlier for your healing)
- Major life changes

These things can take away the balance that you've worked hard to create.

However, you won't be going all the way back to the beginning. You simply need to get back to what you were doing that was working for you.

Be kind to yourself and keep a positive attitude. If you were able to have energy and feel good before you can do it again.

An Opportunity to Grow

Relapse is a common part of any disease and is especially common with chronic fatigue syndrome. But how you view the relapse can help you to recover faster and feel even better than you did before the relapse.

Use this as an opportunity to try and implement more techniques for improving your health. Maybe you haven't tried any forms of massage therapy before, but now might be a good time to see how you can add it to what you're already doing.

Maybe you've improved your diet, but you still eat a lot of refined sugar. A relapse is a good time to focus on adding another component to your plan.

Dropping the sugar could finally help you to have the relief you need for a longer period of time. Adding natural supplements to your nutrition could be the missing ingredient in what you have applied so far in your recovery.

Be Your Own Champion

As you experience the ups and downs of the CFS cycles, you may begin to feel discouraged. But take heart because you have the power to improve your health. You may not have too many people who understand what you're going through.

Having supportive people in your life can be a tremendous help. Sometimes you have to be your own cheerleader and champion as you struggle with this illness.

Supporting Someone with CFS

While someone going through chronic fatigue syndrome is definitely facing challenges, so are the people who support them. It can be difficult to go it alone with this illness and if you have CFS you need all the support you can get.

This chapter is for those of you who love someone or take care of someone with chronic fatigue syndrome.

If you have someone in your life who has chronic fatigue syndrome, this disease affects you, too. There are many things you need to understand so that you can help your loved one and also so that you can gain support.

What You Need to Know

As part of the support system of someone with CFS, there are some things you should know that can help you to understand what's going on. First and foremost, you may want to read this book in its entirety to know more about the symptoms, causes, and treatments for chronic fatigue syndrome.

But just to hit the highlights, there are some critical things that can give you an understanding at-a-glance.

Chronic Fatigue Syndrome is a REAL Illness

While this illness isn't very well understood, it is a real problem. Many people mistakenly believe that chronic fatigue syndrome is just a way to get out of doing your work. In actuality, this is a severe condition that can make it difficult to perform daily tasks or even to do any of the fun things that used to be an enjoyable part of life.

If you have someone who is close to you and supporting you then ask them to read through this list as a starting point to understanding what you are dealing with. After beginning with this overview they should then be encouraged to look through the rest of the book to get a better feel of what you are dealing with.

Someone with chronic fatigue syndrome:

- May appear to look well, even though they're feeling terrible
- Is often experiencing the worst flu like symptoms you could imagine, but having to continue on with their responsibilities
- Has a hard time even completing simple tasks without feeling utterly exhausted
- Needs more rest than other people who don't have CFS
- Have some days with higher energy than others
- Doesn't have an option for a medical cure at this time
- Has constant unexplained aches and pains
- Has trouble sleeping even though exhausted
- Feels depressed because he or she can't have a "normal" life
- Often feels guilty that he or she can't do all the things that once were easy
- Is often harder on herself or himself than you are

As you can imagine this can lead to many feelings such as anger, sadness, and frustration as someone with CFS begins to lose some independence and need more help.

How CFS Can Affect a Caregiver

Someone who has chronic fatigue syndrome is going through major changes. But it's important to remember that it can also mean big changes for the caregivers of that person.

A caregiver helping someone with CFS may be going through:

- Stress of having to take on more household responsibilities
- Financial difficulties because of lost income if the person with CFS can no longer work
- Sadness that the activities you once enjoyed aren't possible at this time
- Fear that your loved one won't get better
- Resentment that the person you're caring for seems to get time for rest and relaxation while you don't have any
- Disbelief that symptoms are as bad as they're reported to be
- Difficulty dealing with personal health issues because of spending time caregiving for someone else
- Physical, mental, and emotional exhaustion
- Frustration with dealing with CFS moodiness or forgetfulness of a loved one

These feelings are natural and normal. You may feel like because you have negative feelings it means you must not love the person you're caring for enough. But that's simply not true.

Being a caregiver for someone with an illness is terribly challenging no matter how much you love him or her. It's important, though, to understand what you're feeling and truly understand the CFS symptoms and progression in order to have some peace.

Tips for Caregivers

In order to become a loving and supportive caregiver without compromising your own health and happiness, there are several things you can do.

Learn All You Can

Many of the problems that plague the relationship between caregivers and those they care for could be solved with understanding. Read as much as you can about chronic fatigue syndrome so that you can understand what your loved one is going through.

Once you see the powerful research and evidence that this is a real problem with real symptoms you'll be able to be more sympathetic to what your loved one is experiencing.

Seek Support

There are support groups for people with CFS and there are also support groups for caregivers. You may want to consider seeking support from one of these groups so that you can find out how other people are learning to cope.

This will give you a safe space to express your feelings, vent your frustrations, and say the things you're afraid to discuss with your loved one.

You may also find that counseling can help you to understand your new role better and a professional can help you to develop a plan that works for you.

Take Care of You

If you don't take care of yourself, you won't have enough energy to help anyone. It's always important to make sure that you're getting enough rest, eating healthy foods, and getting exercise.

You also need to work to reduce your stress levels as much as possible. That may mean that you need to ask other people in your extended circle of family and friends for some help.

It may also mean that you need to let some things go. For example, it's okay if you don't get the floors swept as often as you once did or if the dishes pile up in the sink for a few days. Give yourself permission to take breaks if you need them.

When you feel healthy and whole, you'll be better able to handle the ups and downs of caring for someone with CFS.

Attitude is Everything

Having a negative attitude will attract even more negative energy into your life. It will keep you from being happy and it will make it difficult for someone with CFS to improve. It's important to stay positive.

Looking for the little things in life to be grateful for can be very helpful. It's also helpful to be encouraging to your loved one with CFS. When you notice that he or she is doing well at being consistent with sleep or exercise, make sure to say something positive about it.

When you've had a great day (and there will be great days ahead), take notice of them and enjoy being in the moment. Celebrate every small improvement gained.

Be Flexible

If you become too rigid about your own schedules and plans you'll find that you're often frustrated because of the energy swings caused by CFS. If your loved one needs rest even though you had plans to go out to lunch, try to be flexible and understand that plans need to change.

It's normal to feel disappointed and even angry when things have to change all the time. Bu the more flexible you are, the easier these changes will be for you. When you make plans, just understand that those might have to change.

Don't Become Isolated

When you're caring for someone it's easy to get into a rut of becoming isolated from your regular social group. Make sure to maintain friendships and relationships outside of your household.

Having fun and enjoying time with friends can be the best medicine for someone feeling burned out from caring for someone with a chronic illness.

Don't Take On Extra Responsibilities

When you're caring for someone in the throes of chronic fatigue syndrome, it isn't the time to take on extra responsibilities. Learn to use the word "no" when someone asks you to:

- Head up the carnival at your child's school
- Take on an extra project at work
- Volunteer for the church fundraiser
- Help someone move house
- Babysit, pet sit, or house sit

While it can be hard to say no, people who understand you're having a hard time will accept that you are unable to do any more than you already are juggling.

Don't let anyone make you feel guilty for recognizing and admitting your limitations.

Find New Ways to Share Your Life

While you may not be able to enjoy all the activities that you once did, there can be joy in finding new ways to have fun with your loved one. Finding simple pleasures that make life a little brighter is a way to get through this challenge together.

You need to continue to have fun without spending 100% of your time and energy talking about and dealing with illness. Some ideas for activities with someone who has CFS include:

- Scrapbooking
- Movie marathon at home
- Jigsaw puzzles
- Playing simple games that are slow-paced
- Try takeout from a new restaurant
- Invite a favorite friend over to share dinner or dessert
- Watch or read something funny

Life doesn't always have to be about coping with illness. By finding things to do together that lighten the mood you'll both get benefits.

Be open to trying new things even if they don't seem exciting. They may be just what you need.

Be Kind and Forgiving of Yourself and Others

Being a caregiver for someone with chronic illness is tough. You're going to make mistakes and it's important that you learn to forgive yourself. Constant guilt will only wear you down further.

The other problem you may face is that other people will let you down. You may feel like you need help and don't have the support that you require. Be understanding when other people disappoint you.

And, finally, be understanding of the person you're caring for. Chronic fatigue syndrome is an illness that can be very depressing and frustrating. When your loved one loses his or her temper or is going through negative feelings, try to apply forgiveness and be empathetic.

Know that if they could snap their fingers and make the CFS go away, they wouldn't hesitate.

Dealing with a chronic illness in your household or family is one of the greatest challenges anyone has to face. Don't expect perfection from yourself as you meet these difficulties.

But don't focus so much on the illness you forget to have fun and find the joy in your life. Through some of the greatest trials come the best lessons and the most feelings of fulfillment.

Putting It All Together

Throughout this book we've shared with you many strategies for managing chronic fatigue syndrome. But what works for one person doesn't work for all people.

The idea behind this book is not that you need to do everything in it, but that you need to find what works best for you. Mix and match, combine and test the various therapies and you will eventually find the blend that works best for your recovery.

Be Willing to Try New Things

When you've been newly diagnosed with a chronic illness, everything seems like new and unfamiliar territory. In order to manage your condition you're going to need to be willing to try things you haven't tried before.

Keep a notebook of your experiences so that when something works really well you can continue doing it. And if something doesn't work, you can have a record of why it didn't work and let that idea go.

Don't Put Pressure On Yourself

There are a lot of good ideas here for how you can help get relief from your symptoms. But don't put pressure on yourself to try everything or have expectations about how your recovery and healing will proceed.

Your body is unique and the way that you recover may be different from my experience. That's okay! What's important is to know yourself and pay attention to your own signals and cues.

Don't Delay

Because there is no cure and really not much medical treatment available for CFS, you're going to be highly responsible for your own wellness. The longer you wait to begin taking steps toward a healthier lifestyle, the longer it will take to experience relief.

Get started today by choosing just one thing from this book that you can incorporate into your life right away. Don't get bogged down by thinking you have to do everything in here all at once or do it perfectly every time.

Take a few moments to jot down some changes you've read here that you can implement right now. It may be skipping the coffee or adding a vitamin to your daily routine. It might be taking a nap instead of forcing yourself to keep running on fumes when you ran out of energy long ago today.

Remember That Things Will Get Better

When you're in the beginning or middle of your struggles with CFS it can seem like there's no light at the end of the tunnel. But learning from our experiences and from those of others with CFS that we have helped, there will be a time when things get better for you.

Discouragement can keep you from taking action and make you feel helpless. If you've learned anything by reading the suggestions here, we hope that you've learned that you have a lot of power over your own health and that you can make things better.

It won't happen all at once and it won't happen overnight, but gradually as you learn your own body's triggers and what works for you, you'll gain more energy and start to feel better each day.

We want to thank you for purchasing ***"How to Beat Chronic Fatigue Syndrome and Get Your Life Back!"***

We enjoyed putting this information together for you to give you an overview of Chronic Fatigue Syndrome and to let you get a broad brush picture of what you are dealing with as either a suffer or as a carer of someone who has the condition.

We have endeavored to give you tools to understand your options in how to address your own situation and how to access support from medical and alternative health professionals.

We have indicated areas of alternate healing and given directions as to where to look for more information.

In the future we expect to publish volume 2 of CFS Therapies in a book that that will specifically deal with nutritional and supplementation therapy methods, but within this book we have attempted to deal with the full spectrum of "What is CFS", the medical and non-medical views on the condition and where to go for more information.

We have made every effort to ensure the accuracy and completeness of the content provided in this book.

However, the author or any other person associated with this book makes no warranties or guarantees, expressed or implied, regarding errors or omissions and assumes no legal liability or responsibility for loss or damage resulting from the use of information contained within.

Additionally, the author or associated persons do not guarantee, expressed or implied, for the accuracy, completeness, or usefulness of any information, apparatus, product, or process disclosed, or represents that its use would guarantee improvement or success in relation to subject written.

Any reference herein to any specific commercial products, process, or service by trade name, trademark, manufacturer, or otherwise, does not necessarily constitute or imply its endorsement, recommendation, or favoring.

The content of *"How to Beat Chronic Fatigue Syndrome and Get Your Life Back!"* is copyright protected, with all rights reserved and may not be copied or imitated in whole or part without first requesting and receiving full written permission from the author.

Again, thank you for allowing us to give you this overview on the condition of Chronic Fatigue Syndrome.

If you would like to visit:

http://www.thehealthsuccesssite.com/Chronic-fatigue-syndrome.html you can leave your comments and feedback on this book and ask any questions you may have about CFS in general.

Also we invite you to leave your review of this book at Amazon.

About the Authors

Warren Tattersall

I had a problem with my own health that had plagued me for all of my life.

My elder and younger brothers had high energy levels and I had low energy. I didn't understand why, and I still cannot explain it, but it had been with me all my life and I lived with it.

As a schoolboy I had unexplained energy drop periods where I would just go to bed and sleep for 24 hours. Blood tests showed a drop in the red blood cells in that period but no-one could tell me anything about it.

In my 20's I went to a naturopath to ask about improving energy and she checked my diet and almost had a fit. She had me change my eating process dramatically. I did that for 90 days and it made no difference to the condition at all that I could see.

I had a Homeopathic consultation at one stage and religiously used the drops for a few months in the belief that I needed to stick to anything for at least 90 days. Again, it made not the slightest difference to the way I felt.

I tried a Chinese herbalist once. I figured that anything that tasted that bad HAD to be good for you but again, another 3 months and no energy improvement at all.

When I was going out with the girl who became my wife there was an occasion that I fell asleep while sitting at the table in a restaurant. This is an embarrassing thing at any time but when there are only the 2 of you there is something that keeps being recalled in conversation for 20 years!!

In my early 30's I went to my General Practitioner and had a serious conversation with him because the periods of weariness seemed to be getting worse and I thought there should be something that could be done.

I am 6 ft 2 in (187 cm) and he is much shorter than I am. He did all the blood tests and then patiently explained to me that I was tall and he was short. He did not like being short but there was nothing he could do about it. He said that he had high energy and I had low energy and that was just the way it was. Live with it!!

I'd lived with my 'condition' all my life and after that I pretty much accepted it and I did not really notice the effect of it in my world any more. I just accepted that I naturally had very low energy levels and that every 6 or 8 weeks I would have an energy drop out that would make normal living a big challenge for a few days, but I knew it would pass.

When I started to use the nutritional supplement products from Herbalife it was just to see what it did and because it may be able to give me a benefit for my Martial Arts.

It was only 4 or 5 days later I remember standing at my wardrobe in the morning getting out a shirt and just freezing up. I realized that for the first time in my life I could not remember getting out of bed! I had never just woken up and just got out of bed.

Every day I used to come slowly to consciousness and then fought myself to get moving. This day I just woke up rested and alert. It was one of those moments that you remember forever.

On that day my energy lifted. I can't say it 'came back' because I could never remember having it in the first place. I can miss sleep and get just 4 or 5 hours for a couple of nights in a row and still do not have energy drop-outs during the day. When I do get really tired it is my own fault, but one night with 8 hours sleep and I am refreshed again.

Once I began incorporating these products into my CFS therapy I have not had to do much of anything else, apart from my daily use of nutrition supplements, which is now so engrained into my lifestyle that I do not even notice it.

This has lasted for 20 years now and someone asked me the other day what the side effects are of taking 'supplements' for extended times. In my own case I have an answer to that.

Earlier in the year I turned 55 and as a matter of good practice I occasionally get a full medical check (to be frank the results are always really good so I'm happy to do it).

This last test generated a call from the pathologist re the results and I was concerned that there might be a problem because I had not expected a call. He said that no, quite the reverse.

The results were really good, or at least they would be really good for someone in their mid 20's. He did not believe that results like these, which were uniformly perfect across the full spectrum, were possible for someone in their mid 50's.

The point here is that whatever your personal beliefs may be about the benefits of taking daily supplements and vitamins, it cannot be denied that consistently eating healthy food and supplements has a very positive effect on your body in the long-term.

I think the summary of my own story is that you need to keep looking till you find the answer best suited for you, and when you get it right you can expect, God willing, to regain good health and keep it for decade after decade.

Helene Malmsio

At 17 I was overworked and already anemic, when I contracted glandular fever in 1976. I thought it was just a bad flu and didn't get it treated until my throat was so sore that it was too painful to even take a normal breath.

I did finally get on a course of antibiotics, but did not support my recovery with supplements to help undo the damage of massive doses of antibiotics to my already compromised system, or improve my poor diet.

Sure enough, within a few years I found that I was chronically ill with every cold, flu, allergy, and joint pain that I had ever imagined possible.

Every morning I would wake up feeling like I had the worst Flu ever, multiplied by 10. I also felt a level of total exhaustion like nothing I had ever known before. It was totally bewildering to me.

In 1988 I was laughingly diagnosed with the 'Yuppie Flu' as it was known then, and told to just 'take some rest'. I was running my own business and my workload did not allow for any rest, and within 18 months I was totally incapacitated.

At one point I admit that I even became suicidal from depression and the belief that I would never be able to have a normal life again. There was so much pain and hopelessness, there really did not seem to be anything to look forward to in life.

I was physically incapacitated to the point where I simply could not muster the energy or motivation to get out of bed, never mind to leave the house or go to the office, so I had to close my consulting business.

It required 12 months of bed rest and doing everything I could think of or learn about to help my recovery, before I could muster enough energy to try to participate in the workforce again. My partner at the time informed me that I was the most boring person he knew, because I always had to sleep for the entire weekend just to be able to go back to work again on Monday morning.

In 1991 I found a doctor specializing in CFS treatments who identified 6 common influenza strains in my blood that are known to trigger the illness, along with the initial GF. He said that he was surprised I was able to function at all, never mind be able to hold down a job, as my case was one of the most severe he had seen.

I was prescribed a 90 day CFS treatment program that included a range of dozens of bottles of Vega tested vitamins and minerals to take every day, with half a dozen oral allergy drops to build my immunity to these triggers also attacking my system.

And every week I endured an hour of an IV feeding a vitamin mix direct into my blood and organs. This treatment would then send my body into a state of shock for the rest of the day, with shivering and considerable pain throughout my entire body. And I achieved absolutely no relief from my CFS at the end of the long treatment program.

My doctor told me that I should just try undertaking another course of the same treatment. I felt shattered and hopeless again, as I simply could not endure another few months of that painful treatment.

But I was on a cause, and determined to get my life back. I kept researching and testing. And as a result of spending the last 25 years checking out every possible therapy I have ever heard of, I now know how to cope better with my CFS and how to recover from relapses when they happen.

As a result I now know how to pace myself, and how to deal with the cyclical relapses, what nutritional supplements work for me, and I still apply a combination of the therapies featured in this book for an individual CFS therapy plan that works for me.

Nowadays I am often even considered to be a 'dynamic' person by some people, and that is a testament to how well you can recover under the right circumstances.

My hope is that sharing this information in this book set will be of help to you and save you many years of experimenting and testing like I had to undergo. I really look forward to publishing the second book in this series, as I believe you will get as much benefit as I have from applying nutritional supplementation therapy to beat your CFS.

Check out the next page for a preview of our next book in this series:

"Nutritional Therapy Guide for a CFS Diet …how to eat yourself healthy again"

Chapter One:
What is Chronic Fatigue Syndrome?
The Basics of this Condition

Chronic Fatigue Syndrome, or CFS, is a condition that plagues millions of people worldwide. Imagine feeling as if you have the flu and have such fatigue that you're unable to carry out your normal activities. Worse, imagine being so fatigued all the time that you just cannot get up and function normally and you can only get out of bed for a couple of hours a day.

People all across the world are living with this condition. If you are one of them we hope we can guide you to be able to turn around your condition and to feel well again.

If you have someone you know who suffers with CFS, or has symptoms similar to the ones related here, then this book should give you an insight into their world, how they feel, and give you some practical strategies to help support them to deal with their condition.

Normally, with CFS, when you go to the doctor, you don't have any specific illness that can be diagnosed and no one seems to understand how truly terrible you feel. Those who battle CFS can feel this way for months at a time.

In some cases the CFS condition seems to take over people's lives and they can lose not months, but years, of healthy living. These people are often young and often fit athletes and high performers in their field before they are stuck down by CFS.

In this section we'll outline some of the basic information about chronic fatigue symptoms and causes that are detailed further in the main body of this book, as well as the recommended methods of using nutritional therapy within a healing CFS diet.

CFS Symptoms

Chronic Fatigue Syndrome can be experienced in different ways. But the basic symptoms are:

Tiredness – extreme tiredness that isn't relieved after rest
Headaches – chronic headaches
Sleep problems – either you can't sleep or sleep doesn't bring rest
Muscle pain – pain that can't be explained by recent activities

These are the hallmark symptoms of the condition. But you may notice from this list that these symptoms could be part of other illnesses. It's important that if you suspect you have CFS that you speak with your doctor.

CFS is diagnosed if the above symptoms are present for a period of six months and there is an absence of another health condition. You'll need to make sure and rule out other illnesses that can cause these symptoms.

You may also experience other symptoms along with the main ones, including:

Food allergies and intolerances
Chronic tiredness that keeps people in bed much of the day and that requires regular naps to prevent the sufferer falling asleep as they try to undertake normal activities
Chronic diarrhea
Chronic sore throat
Night sweats
Weight loss
Nausea
Dizziness
Shortness of breath

For people with advanced CFS we do not need to list their symptoms as they are all too familiar with them but ultimately some people develop sensitivity to environmental conditions that can prevent them from living in normal modern society.

Many other symptoms may apply to your specific case of Chronic Fatigue Syndrome. It's important to remember that this condition is very individual so you may have symptoms that others don't.

How Will CFS Impact Your Life?

Many people have trouble keeping up with their regular activities when they have CFS. You may feel like you just need to stay in bed and aren't able to go to work.

Many people find that they can't do many of the things they once enjoyed or that they cannot find the motivation to get started to get out undertaking these things. They just cannot get themselves moving.

What's worse, with CFS many people other people who see you with these symptoms don't understand that you have a real health condition. They may not understand why you can't work or they may feel frustrated that you're not able to continue old activities. This is often especially true for those who are closest to you.

Some people battle CFS for a few months and then get better, never having a relapse. But for many people there are cycles of fatigue followed by feeling better, then dealing with a frustrating return of fatigue.

Others seem to have these cycles but the fatigue level keeps getting deeper each time till they fall into a condition where they cannot even function in normal daily routines.

This can go on for a few years before the body is able to say goodbye to CFS and some people even deal with it over a lifetime. But with good therapy, particularly in the area of nutrition, you can turn around your condition and experience healing and once again feel better health.

What Causes CFS?

If you have chronic fatigue, you no doubt want to find out the cause. Unfortunately, there is no formal recognition of a specific cause of CFS yet. There are a few theories out there though:

The most common scientific theory is that CFS is caused by a virus that you've contracted at some point in your life.

We will talk later about the root cause potentially being an issue with your body's ingestion of nutrition. That is often brought on through lifestyle factors, high stress, and often seems to be linked to the use of antibiotics.

Others still seem to have a problem that has a foundation involving chemicals contamination and having residual chemicals in their body.

All of these paths to the condition seem to manifest in slightly different ways. The path out of them can also vary depending on the underlying issues but, in practical terms, the end result of how people feel and function when they are suffering with CFS seems to follow a similar pattern no matter what the cause.

Chronic Fatigue Syndrome has probably been around for centuries, but it's only been in the last century that it's gotten attention. And only in the last couple of decades has it been recognized as a true medical problem.

While CFS was once thought to be a psychological problem, in the past decade it's been seen by the medical community as a real illness. This has led to more research. While, as we said, there's no formally recognized cause yet, there are scientists hard at work looking to identify one and to better understand the condition.

The problem that faces people with CFS is that since no formally recognized cause has been identified this flows through to a situation where there isn't a medically recognized targeted medication, formalized treatment procedure, or cure for Chronic Fatigue Syndrome. It would be wonderful if you could get a prescription that would take care of CFS for good, but that's just not something available right now.

That is why this book covers alternative health information that does not claim to provide a cure but that has been shown to guide people back on to the path of healing and improved health.

We know that there are some things that can contribute to the development of CFS in the body as well as to other disease. Much of it has to do with our modern lifestyle and environmental stress that our lives place on us.

We expect that you will find some very logical and helpful answers for your own situation as we look at these things together and look at potential options, especially nutritional supplementation, to help deal with these things

For example, we're exposed to many more toxins nowadays than we have been exposed to in the past. Toxins can be found in the pollution in the air we breathe, contamination in the ground we walk on, and in more and more in the food that we eat. The more we're exposed to these toxins the more strain we place on the immune system.

In addition, the modern Western diet contains many processed grains and refined sugars that are also unhealthy for the body. And we don't get enough of the good, healthy foods we need.

Having a high stress lifestyle and broken sleep patterns can also cause the body to break down its immunity. A busy schedule coupled with lack enough sleep, or irregular sleep, can magnify the problem that stress creates for the body.

We will look at how all these things can come together into a crisis for your body. This can lead to an event, or series of events, in life being a trigger point where people see their CFS condition as starting.

There are also more substances that are taken such as prescription medication, alcohol, and other illicit drugs that can break down your body's ability to fight infection and illness.

In thinking about your own lifestyle, you may be able to identify some factors that have led to your body's breakdown. But it's important not to dwell on the past and just make the decision to work at improvement from this day forward.

We will take time review the past with you though so you can see a path forward. We will then show you tools to deal with your situation and to get you moving back to health and to an active lifestyle.

Printed in Germany
by Amazon Distribution
GmbH, Leipzig